SH*T
I WISHED I
KNEW BEFORE I
DISCHARGED

DAN PRONK

**To find out more about this book or
to contact the author, please visit:
www.vividpublishing.com.au/danpronk**

Copyright © 2024 Dan Pronk

ISBN: 978-1-923078-14-7
Published by Vivid Publishing
A division of Fontaine Publishing Group
P.O. Box 948, Fremantle
Western Australia 6959
www.vividpublishing.com.au

NATIONAL LIBRARY OF AUSTRALIA A catalogue record for this
book is available from the
National Library of Australia

CONTENTS

1. You may not see the cliff coming

I had thought I'd seen the cliff coming for six months before I eventually fell off it, and I felt that I had prepared myself well.

I was wrong.

Having spent the preceding 14 years in the army, the last five of which with special operations, I was looking forward to a slower-paced and simpler life with my young family. As a doctor, job prospects post-army were good and promised wages significantly higher than what I had been earning during my military service. We would be moving back to a newly built house in my wife's hometown which meant more social support for the family, and I had accumulated a significant amount of leave which would allow me to ease back into a civilian life without the pressure of needing to immediately find work. As a precaution to stave off boredom and to have a structured focus in my life following my immediate discharge, I had enrolled in a Master of Business Administration online.

I was physically relatively uninjured from my service,

and while I had experienced a significant degree of psychological trauma during my four tours of Afghanistan with
Special Operations, at that point I was seemingly largely un-
affected by symptoms of Post-Traumatic Stress. I had naïvely
anticipated that the void that would be created in my life by
leaving the army could be neatly filled by increased family
time, post-graduate study, a new job, and increased income.

Within six months of transition from army to civilian
life the cracks were well and truly beginning to appear in
the armour. Demons from my service, centred primarily on
the memories of soldiers I couldn't save, began to infiltrate
my conscious thoughts, and caused my palms to sweat and
my heart to race. My sleep was regularly disturbed by vivid
dreams of my family members drowning and me not being
able to save them despite my best efforts. Crowded places
caused me to become highly anxious and the smell of raw
pork started making me gag.

As a doctor I of course recognised these symptoms as
those of Post-Traumatic Stress (PTS), it just seemed odd
that they were occurring at a time when I was safer than
ever, home more than ever, and earning more money than
ever. Surely, you'd think those symptoms should have been
happening in the thick of it, when I was being regularly
exposed to stressful situations and trauma. It got me
reflecting deeply on what the protective factors were at
the time when I was in the army, that allowed me to stay
resilient despite the stress and exposures. What metaphoric
armour had I lost when I took off my literal armour for the

last time and walked away from the military? Maybe if I could figure that out it would provide a roadmap of sorts back to a resilient version of myself as a civilian[1].

As time progressed, I became convinced that PTS was only a small component of what was at play. As I reintegrated into the workforce as a fly-in, fly-out doctor on a mine site it became clear that the process that had derailed my life was as much a grief response as it was PTS.

I was grieving the person I used to be and had absolutely no idea how to be the new person that I had become. I had lost my identity. I was grieving the loss of my previous army support structure, who I had shared experiences with and who truly understood me. I had lost my tribe.

I had hopped off the fast-moving army special operations train and my pace of life had slowed abruptly. I felt unsettled and unstimulated. I was bored shitless. I felt a cavernous divide between me and the civilians that now surrounded me, with no obvious way for me to traverse that divide and become one of them. Furthermore, I had absolutely no desire to become one of them; I was caught between worlds with seemingly no way back and no way forward.

All of this was happening in the context of me discharging from the army by my own choice, in relatively good physical and mental health, with an intact marriage and loving family, and having a qualification as a doctor that translated perfectly into civilian life.

---

[1] Opening vignette is taken from Chapter 1 of Pronk D, Pronk B, and Curtis T, 2021, *The Resilience Shield*, Macmillan Australia, Sydney.

On paper everything was perfect, yet from a mental health perspective I was doing worse than I ever had been. It just didn't seem right. I knew there must be a pathway back to a resilient and thriving version of myself, I'd been that person before, and I was confident I could be that person again. I just needed a roadmap to get there.

My initial attempts to cope consisted of the predictable maladaptive practices of pouring alcohol on my demons and training physically until exhaustion. On several occasions, I found myself collapsed next to the punching bag in my shed, having thumped it with bare knuckles until my hands were covered in blood in a futile attempt to release the rage that seemed to be constantly lurking just beneath the surface of my consciousness.

At around the six-month mark post discharge and strongly encouraged by my wife, who could see the changes in me, I attended my one and only appointment with a Veteran's Affairs psychologist.

I'm not sure if what I recall of that session was what actually happened, or if it was coloured by my mental state at the time, but it wasn't what I was hoping for. After providing a brief overview of my experiences, including responding to multiple teammates of mine on the battlefield who I couldn't save, the psychologist basically concluded that PTSD was the issue, and the next priority was for me to see one of the department's psychiatrists for a formal diagnosis. There was talk of pensions and medications, but I had switched off. I had gone to the psychologist for tools, not a diagnosis. I had wanted to assemble a team of professionals around me to support me in finding my path back to a thriving version of myself, not a team to diagnose and medicate me.

I left the psychologist's office that day and never went back.

Embarrassingly, on reflection, I can now see that part of my reluctance to be formally diagnosed with PTSD was due to the stigma associated with the diagnosis, compounded by fear of what it would mean for my medical registration as a practicing doctor to have a mental health diagnosis.

But it was more than that.

While I was certain that my symptoms were consistent with Post-Traumatic Stress, I didn't feel that I had had them long enough to resign myself to having a *disorder*. Part of me feared that acceptance of the diagnosis by formalising it might lead to me, consciously or subconsciously, adopting it as my new identity. I feared developing a victim mentality.

More than that though, I could see clearly that the PTS symptoms were only a fraction of my troubles at the time. The larger part was what the psychologists call *adjustment disorder*, intensified by the unique stresses that come from leaving a high-performance, tight knit organisation such as the military. I would later learn of the concept of *transition stress*[2], which beautifully encompasses everything I was experiencing at the time.

---

[2] I first heard this term in Mobbs, M. C., & Bonanno, G. A. (2018). "Beyond war and PTSD: The crucial role of transition stress in the lives of military veterans": Corrigendum. *Clinical Psychology Review, 60*, 147.

I've titled this book "Shit I wished *I* knew before I discharged" for a reason. It is based on *my* personal experiences, observations, perspectives, and trial and error. It is the roadmap that I eventually assembled to start, slowly but surely, rebuilding myself as a civilian after discharge.

It is not designed to be a one-size-fits-all program for every transitioning military, police, and emergency services member, rather it is designed to seed thoughts and stimulate reflection and consideration about the psychological factors at play during transition and hopefully provide a small amount of light to illuminate the path out of the dark space that can follow transition. That path need only be illuminated a few steps ahead at any given time and it will take years to walk fully out of the darkness into the light of a post-transition life, but it is possible.

Like any challenge we faced in our previous professional roles, there is always a solution, and that solution starts with a good understanding of the problem we're dealing with.

A quote that resonates deeply with me and that I feel is relevant here comes from the book *Green Lights* by Matthew McConaughey[3]:

"Once you know it's black, it's not near as dark"

This book is designed to help understand the problem of transition because, once you know it's black, it's not near as dark. This metaphor highlights the requirement to define what we're up against in the transition process. In effect, to know our enemy. But there's more than that; we also need to

---

[3] McConaughy, M, 2020, *Green Lights*, Headline, New York.

truly know ourselves. As the great Sun Tzu offers us in *The Art of War*[4]:

> If you know the enemy and know yourself, you need not fear the result of a hundred battles.
>
> If you know yourself but not the enemy, for every victory gained you will suffer a defeat.
>
> If you know neither the enemy nor yourself, you will succumb to every battle.

I fear that many transitioning military members and first responders succumb to the battle due to not having the tools to truly reflect and know themselves, and not having a deep understanding of the psychological enemy that they're battling in transition. Hopefully this book will help.

The first thing to realise is that transition is going to suck! Let's have a look at why.

---

[4] Tzu, S, 2017, *The Art of War*, Arcturus, London.

2. Transition is going to suck.

As mentioned in Chapter 1, I hadn't anticipated the fact that transition was going to suck. I certainly hadn't appreciated that it was going to suck hard and for years and years!

As pessimistic as it might sound, I think that adopting a mindset that transition is going to suck is useful, as it primes you to be ready for the challenge. Perhaps even to *embrace the suck!*

I appreciate that my experience was fortunate in the fact that I discharged from the army at a time of my own choosing with an intact family unit, good health, and good job prospects. I have witnessed plenty of my mates transition with far worse social, mental, physical, emotional, and professional situations than mine and can only imagine the amplification of the transition stress under those circumstances.

One of the traps that I can now see I fell into in the lead up to transition was looking ahead and only seeing the positives. In my last six months with the army, I had become a bit stale in my role and with hindsight (although I didn't realise it at the time) was burnt out. For the first time in my military career, I had started to focus intently on the negatives of the job and, when thinking about discharge, was experiencing what is known as *confirmation bias*, being the tendency to interpret new information and evidence as confirmation of our existing beliefs.

I had made the decision to discharge from the army, so I was starting to see all the evidence that helped justify my decision and confirm it as the correct one. Confirmation bias can help us feel better about our decisions but can blind us to a balanced perspective of things. In my instance, I suspect it contributed to my complete inability to see or consider the negative aspects of leaving the army.

I'm going to take a deep dive into all the factors that I feel led to my struggles in transition in chapters to come, but as an overview the key ones are as follows:

- Loss of Identity and Grieving my former self
- Loss of Tribe and feelings of Loneliness
- Loss of Motivation and Purpose
- Loss of Self Esteem
- Slowing of my pace of life and feeling Bored Shitless

I can now see that it was a combination of all the above factors that led to a significant drop in my overall resilience, allowing the cumulative stress and unprocessed traumatic exposures of my military service to finally catch up with me and kick me in the arse!

While this all seems like doom and gloom, when I

started to realise the psychological factors at play during transition (this took years to do!), I started to see a glimpse of the roadmap out of the dark space. I could see that the way to rebuild myself was to deliberately recreate the factors in my life that I had shed in transition from the military.

My mind works in a very scientific way and for that reason I turned to the psychological literature to provide me with the evidence I needed to understand what was happening and to serve as a starting point to formulating my roadmap forward. This was what I had been hoping to get from the psychologist when I had my one and only visit but didn't.

Hands-down, the best article I came across on the topic was written by Meaghan Mobbs and George Bonanno and is titled *Beyond war and PTSD: The crucial role of transition stress in the lives of military veterans*[5].

While the article takes the perspective of the transitioning military veteran, in my opinion the concepts are directly applicable to anyone transitioning out of roles including policing, emergency services such as firefighters and paramedics, correctional staff, and the list goes on. Basically, anyone who has been indoctrinated into a role that is high stress, has unique exposures not common in more *normal* jobs, and who has integrated into a tight knit *tribe* of people with shared experiences and suffering.

[5] Mobbs, M. C., & Bonanno, G. A. (2018). "Beyond war and PTSD: The crucial role of transition stress in the lives of military veterans": Corrigendum. *Clinical Psychology Review, 60*, 147.

Mobbs & Bonanno address the very real issue of PTSD in the veteran population but point out statistics supporting the fact that, depending on the study cited, on average only 10% of Iraq and Afghanistan veterans suffer from PTSD (accepting that many veterans who might meet a formal diagnosis of PTSD don't seek support due to the many barriers that exist).

Now, this isn't for one minute designed to diminish the experience of those veterans with a PTSD diagnosis. PTSD is very real, can be debilitating, and deserves the rightful attention it gets, and the resources allocated to helping those with the diagnosis. What is interesting however is the research also cited in Mobbs & Bonanno that:

> "...44% to 77% of veterans experience high levels of stress during the transition to civilian life, including difficulties during employment, conflicted relations with family, friends, and broader interpersonal relations, difficulties adapting to the schedule of civilian life, and legal difficulties."

Muddying the waters here is that transition stress and Post-Traumatic Stress can, and often do, coexist. I strongly suspect that this was the case in my instance, with the stress of transition lowering my resilience and causing symptoms of PTS to emerge. However, looking at the statistics above, there is a definite disconnect between PTSD diagnosis statistics and the percentage of veterans experiencing high levels of stress during transition from military life.

From my observations, much of the psychological support available to veterans is linked to a diagnosis of PTSD and I wonder how many have been stamped with that diagnosis (with the best of intentions) to allow them to access services, when what they were actually experiencing was primarily transition stress. The mental health and professional implications of a formal diagnosis of PTSD can be significant and might perhaps have been avoidable in some instances, it's impossible to say.

Just how much transition is going to suck and for how long is a very individual thing and is impossible to predict with complete accuracy for any single person. Even under my somewhat ideal circumstances I would say that my transition to feeling like a properly thriving civilian after my time in the army took around 5-6 years. That said, I think there are some rough rules of thumb that can be applied, starting with this basic equation:

Suckiness of Transition = Time in Role x Investment in Role

This make sense, right? If we use the analogy of an intimate interpersonal relationship, we can see some parallels. If you have a one-night stand with a partner then never see them again, then it's unlikely to derail your life as the relationship was fleeting and a deep connection probably wasn't established.

At the other end of the spectrum, if you've been in a

long-term relationship with someone, perhaps married, and have started to build a life together, then the difficulty of that breakup is likely to cause significant stress and pain. If you have kids together then of course that compounds the suckiness of the situation. The circumstances of the breakup will also influence the stress of the situation. For example, if your intimate partner has cheated on you then that is going to be even more traumatic than an amicable separation.

The same principles apply when considering the level of suckiness of transitioning from a military or emergency services role. If you've done a couple of years as a volunteer firefighter then as a generalisation the transition process should be easier to negotiate than a career police officer who entered the police academy at age 17, rose through the ranks, and then was forced into retirement at age 65.

Likewise, if you transition by your own choice and with good career prospects (as I did) then that should be an easier process to negotiate than if you were forced to discharge for physical health, mental health, or disciplinary reasons, and maybe don't have a skillset that translates well into life after service in your previous role.

The duration of service and investment in a role are key factors that will influence the suckiness of the transition period, but there's more to it than that. Listed below are some other factors that are likely to either compound the difficulty, or potentially be protective, during transition.

Factors compounding Suckiness of Transition

- Entry into role at a younger age – ie: straight out of school
- Transition for involuntary reasons, such as:
  o medical or psych discharge
  o disciplinary or administrative causes
  o mandatory retirement due to age when you didn't feel ready to leave.
- Physical or mental injury from your service
- Lack of formal qualifications that translate beyond your previous role
- Lack of friendships outside of work tribe
- Lack of interests outside of work

Factors reducing Suckiness of Transition

- Life/work experience prior to entry into role
- Voluntary transition from role
- Formal qualifications that allow meaningful employment following transition
- Friendships outside of work tribe
- Interests outside of work
- Established relationships with a General Practitioner (Family Doctor), psychologist, and/or counsellor outside of work

Call to action: calculate your Transition Suck Factor (TSF).

For all the factors in the left column pick the category that describes you best and add up your TSF points.

	1 Point	2 Points	3 Points
Years of service	<10	10-20	>20
Investment in Service	It was just a job	I quite liked it	I lived and breathed it
Age on entry into the role	>30 years old	20-30 years old	<20 years old
Did you transition by your own choice?	Yes		No
Are you physically or mentally injured from your service?	No significant physical or mental injuries	A few bangs and bruises	Significant physical and/or mental injuries from service
Do you have skills or qualifications that translate well post-transition?	Skills and qualifications translate directly to get meaningful work	Skills and qualifications translate ok – should be able to get work	Skills and qualifications don't translate well to get meaningful work
How many close friends (including family) do you have outside of work?	4 or more	1-3	0

How many interests or hobbies do you have outside of work?	2 or more	1	0
Do you have established relationships with a General Practitioner (Family Doctor) and/or a psychologist/counsellor outside of work?	Established contact with specialists you trust	Aware of specialists you feel you could build a relationship with	None

Scoring

TSF <12: You're in good shape! Transition will still likely be stressful, but you've got a bunch of strong positive factors on your side to power on with life.

TSF 13-20: This is going to be a rocky road, but you've got some good protective factors on your side

TSF >21: There's no sugar-coating the fact, transition is probably going to be a very difficult time. But don't despair, this book is all about helping you through it!

Obviously, the TSF scale is a bit tongue-in-cheek and

doesn't consider all the factors that influence the transition experience. Its purpose is to get you thinking about some of the key determinants that influence the difficulty of the transition period. The goal is to begin to demystify why transition is so stressful to know the enemy that you need to fight and give you the best chance of winning.

In my opinion, one of the fundamental factors that causes stress in transition is the loss of identity that comes with moving out of a military, police, or other first responder role.

To grasp the magnitude of the impact of identity loss, it's useful to go back to the start of a career and explore how that identity is formed in the first place. Having an insight into identity formation provides clues as to how to rebuild a positive new identity post-transition. Let's jump into that discussion in the next chapter.

3. You will lose your identity

When I reflect on my own experience of transition, I think at the very core of my transition stress was my near-complete loss of identity when I left the army. It was something I hadn't even considered, and it left me feeling completely lost.

Most of us don't give any deep consideration to our identity, or to the factors that contributed to its formation. If you've progressed along a somewhat normal childhood and adolescent trajectory, then your identity gradually forms along the way without much conscious thought. You just become who you are and if that is an acceptable outcome then you don't have cause to consider or challenge it. If it ain't broke, don't fix it!

To better understand the abrupt loss of identity that most feel on transition from military or emergency services roles I think it's useful to take a deeper dive into how identity in general, and specifically the *role identity* that follows, is formed.

Let's start with a dictionary definition of identity. The

Oxford Dictionary defines identity as:

> "A phenomenological sense of oneself as a separate being with a distinctive personality and a 'true self' persisting over time; a self-image".

Ignoring the wanky use of the word *phenomenological*, the key things here are our *distinctive true self* and the *persistence* of this over time.

There are a bunch of models describing how we form our identities, but one of the gurus on the topic was the German American developmental psychologist, Erik Erikson.

Erikson focused on the adolescent period as a fundamental point in our identity development. He described this as a period of *identity crisis* when the questions of "who am I?" and "who do I want to be?" weigh heavily on us.

During this period, we're experimenting with different identities to see which one fits (for me, this included a period of having dreadlocks and an earring, which thankfully didn't stick!) and exploring what suits us with regards to appearance, education, vocational choices and aspirations, relationships, sexuality, social and political views, personality, and interests.

Once we've tried on a few different identities, and often heavily influenced by external reactions and influences at the time, most of us eventually resolve this identity crisis and reach what Erikson termed *identity achievement*.

Another renowned researcher in the identity space is James Marcia, who elaborated on Erikson's work and describes the situation that occurs when Erikson's identity crisis is not resolved in adolescence.

Marcia used the term *identity diffusion* to describe adolescents who have neither explored the options, nor made a commitment to an identity. Those who persist in this state tend to drift aimlessly with little connection to people around them and have little sense of purpose in life.

Adolescents experiencing identity diffusion are often passive, living in the moment, and have little consideration of who they are or who they want to be. Their primary goals can gravitate towards the short-term seeking of pleasure and avoidance of pain. They're externally oriented, have low levels of autonomy, take less personal responsibility for their lives, and may feel isolated and withdrawn from the world.

Back to Erikson, he proposed that one's occupation and one's commitment to certain values and beliefs are fundamental components of identity.

It is often around the late adolescent stage, when an individual is achieving their adult identity, that it is also time to start looking for a career. For those who gravitate towards jobs such as military, policing, and other first responder roles, this is often the age when they will enter the training pipeline for those professions. As such, they are heavily influenced by the organisational values and beliefs of those professional organisations at a time when they are solidifying their adult identity. Hence, they can form their first adult identity *as* a member of that organisation.

The nature of the training pipelines for military and

emergency responder roles can serve to intensify this identity formation through the relative isolation from broader society during training, as well as the unique and intensive nature of the training itself.

All going well, the individual is learning and growing at a rapid rate and feeling the sense of self accomplishment that comes with meeting the difficult assessment criteria required to progress to qualification in the role. Their individual adult identity is being solidified in the context of the organisational values and beliefs and more than that, they are being bonded together through mutual suffering with others undergoing the same hardships. A strong sense of *social identity* and the beginnings of a tribal affiliation with other trainees has begun (more on that in the next chapter).

A powerful comment which describes this period from a US military perspective can be found in Mobbs & Bonanno's article (which if you haven't read yet, you must):

"The crucible of entry level training is meant to strip away the vestiges of the civilian identity and transform men and women into Soldiers, Sailors, Airmen, and Marines".

Although police, firefighters, paramedics, correctional officers, and other first responders remain civilians by definition, the very same process is at play with them being indoctrinated into an organisation and tribe that, in my opinion, is distinctly different from the broader civilian population.

As the individual enters the workforce in their role and gains further experience and competence, their individual and group identities are further solidified. This provides the *persistence over time* aspect that is crucially important to a stable identity.

Drawing from other models of identity (of which there are many), further key elements include a sense of significance and purpose. It's easy to see how these elements are positively reinforced in military and first responder roles. The longer an individual remains in their role, and barring something unforeseen, the stronger their identity becomes. All going well, this is a positive thing, right up until the point of transition…

Having discussed the frictions of identity development in adolescence, it can be seen that the transitioning military member or first responder gets thrust straight back into a state of identity crisis, with the question evolving from the original "who am I?" to "who am I *now*?".

Once again, this identity crisis needs to be resolved to reach the point of a new identity achievement. This can be a far more difficult proposition the second time around, particularly if the individual has spent years or decades as their old identity, and moreso if they loved that identity. The *persistence over time* aspect that is crucial to, and forms part of the dictionary definition of identity, is abruptly broken.

Just like the adolescent trying on different identities until they find one that fits, the transitioning member needs to do the same. Just like the adolescent spending years testing and adjusting their identity, the transitioning member needs to appreciate that new identity formation is not going to be a quick process. There will be ups and downs, trial, and error, and it will take years to reach a new state of identity achievement. Care needs to be taken to ensure that this new identity is a positive one! Effort also needs to be made to avoid a prolonged period of Marcia's *identity diffusion* characterised by lack of commitment to a new identity, lack of purpose and direction, and disconnection with those around them.

This process is challenging enough for those members (like me) who transition on their own terms. I can only imagine that it is exponentially more difficult for those who are forced into transition involuntarily through medical or psychological injury. In this setting, another aspect of identity is at play, known as *disability identity*.

Disability Identity in the unique aspect of identity that includes a person's sense of self as someone with a disability, as well as their connection with the disability community. For a formerly high functioning military member or first responder, this can be overwhelmingly confronting. To go from the heights of their operational capacity to identifying as a person with a disability is understandably often devastating to their sense of self and is predictably one of the barriers to individuals seeking out a formal diagnosis of physical and mental health injuries, and thus preventing them from accessing the optimal care for those conditions. It is just too foreign a concept to accept themselves as *disabled* as it is in direct opposition to their former sense of being a purposeful member of their organisation and doing something of significance. The transition from being the person who answers calls for help, to the person who asks for help, is often psychologically insurmountable (I'll pick up on this topic again in Chapter 5).

Factors making up our identity

Many aspects of our adult identity are relatively fixed and, while they might play a small role in the transition process, probably aren't going to influence it significantly. These aspects include:

- Gender
- Sex
- Sexual orientation
- Race
- Ethnicity
- Social class
- Religion
- Citizenship and nationality
- Ancestry
- Physical appearance
- Birth order
- Languages spoken
- Caste status
- Political views

Other aspects of identity are highly relevant to transition and a bit of time spent drilling down into them can be instrumental in helping with resolving the identity crisis that comes with transition and the achievement of a new identity. These include:

- Personality
- Profession (former)
- Skills
- Hobbies
- Values

Call to action: Know thyself!

Personality

If you haven't done any personality profiling, or haven't done it recently, it's worth doing one or more of the many available tests to get a good idea of your personality. This can be informative in gaining insight into who you are at the time of transition and thus aligning the direction you head in search of your new identity in accordance with what suits your personality.

All the personality tests have their fans and critics and none of them should be taken as a definitive diagnostic for your personality. That said, a few that I consider useful are:

- Myers-Briggs Type Indicator
- Big Five Assessment
- DiSC

Whack those into google, or more broadly search for "personality tests" and you'll usually be able to find some free tests to get you going.

Professional qualifications / Skills

Take some time to reflect on what professional qualifications you have earned in your former role, as well as the skills that you have gained that may not be reflected in formal qualifications.

Often in military and first responder roles individuals gain skills in things like leadership and crisis management that they take for granted but that aren't always assumed knowledge in broader civilian roles and organisations. Mapping your professional qualifications and skills is a great starting point to look for future employment to build a new profession that will contribute to a positive new identity. If your transition is due to reaching retirement age, this process is still useful to look at what you could uniquely offer the broader community in realms such as volunteer work, teaching, or mentoring, all of which can provide significant fulfilment and contribute to a positive identity.

Professional Qualifications	Skills

Hobbies

Your hobbies are another great area to consider in transition. This may mean hobbies that you've continued through your former career or perhaps hobbies you once enjoyed but that have fallen away due to the time commitments of your work. Hobbies can potentially provide clues to what new work role you might find stimulating, or perhaps even something you can develop into a side-hustle or small business idea. Even in the absence of the ability to monetise your hobbies, they can be a great way to diffuse stress and tap into cathartic flow states (more on those later) to be a better version of yourself during transition.

Work/Side-Hustle Hobbies	Hobbies just for Fun and Flow

Values

Most of us inherently know what our personal values are but, like our personality, a lot of us don't take the time to define them or consider them deeply. Knowing what you value with clarity can be a guiding light towards what career or other endeavours you will find fulfilling post-transition. A good place to start is by having a look at the list of common values below[6] and see what resonates with you.

• Authenticity	• Creativity	• Justice	• Religion
• Achievement	• Curiosity	• Kindness	• Respect
• Adventure	• Determination	• Knowledge	• Responsibility
• Authority	• Fairness	• Leadership	• Security
• Autonomy	• Faith	• Learning	• Self-Respect
• Balance	• Fame	• Love	• Service
• Beauty	• Friendships	• Loyalty	• Spirituality
• Boldness	• Fun	• Meaningful Work	• Stability
• Compassion	• Growth	• Openness	• Success
• Challenge	• Happiness	• Optimism	• Status
• Citizenship	• Honesty	• Peace	• Trustworthiness
• Community	• Humour	• Pleasure	• Wealth
• Competency	• Influence	• Popularity	• Wisdom
• Contribution	• Inner Harmony	• Recognition	

I recommend you write those values down (next to the results from your personality tests and your list of professional qualifications and skills!).

For us to be happy it's very important to be acting in accordance with our values. This extends to the workplace, ideally being in a role with organisational values that align with our personal values. The failure to achieve this is what

[6] List adapted from: https://jamesclear.com/core-values

the psychologists call *value incongruence* and leads to an often subconscious feeling of unease or dissatisfaction at work.

One point to consider here is that the values that served you well in your former military or first responder role may not necessarily serve you well moving forward in a new professional role, or in life in general. I'll talk further about the potential need to change your values slightly on transition (based on my own difficult lessons learned) in Chapter 11, but for now it's all about mapping your current values.

The tool that I recommend is *The Values Project* run by the University of Western Australia. At the time of writing, their survey can be found at www.thevaluesproject.com and in under 10 minutes it will give you a detailed analysis of your current values. It's important to answer the survey honestly and not in a manner that you think will give you the best results!

My Current Values

There are no right and wrong values, simply those that you rate more highly than others. Everyone is different, which is part of what makes life so fun. Getting an accurate idea of your current values is another excellent insight into how best to negotiate transition in a manner that is congruent with what you value.

In this chapter we've concentrated on individual identity, however themes of another aspect of identity have started to emerge, that being social identity. Our identity is made up not only of the sense of who we are as individuals but also as who we are as a member of social groups.

Social identity is a massive part of membership to a military or first responder tribe and is the topic of the next chapter.

4. You will lose your tribe

I think that the term *tribe* describes the sense of social interaction and support that I felt with my military colleagues
perfectly. My tribe consisted of others that I would literally
risk my life to help if they were in need and I knew they
would do the same for me.

Outside of family groups, probably the only other
realms where this sort of bond is seen are military and
first responder communities (and perhaps some realms of
adventure sports such as the climbing community). I can't
speak with authority, but I wouldn't expect to find this sort
of tribal bond and willingness to sacrifice for one another in
the average office job or retail store.

The author, Sebastian Junger, captures the essence of
this bond in military members in his book titled *Tribe: On
Homecoming and Belonging*. Junger also has a powerful
TED talk titled *Why veterans miss war* that speaks to this
tribal affiliation as well as broader topics relevant to transition[7]. While Junger's work is centred around the military,

---

[7] https://www.ted.com/talks/sebastian_junger_why_veterans_miss_
war?language=en

the themes are once again highly relevant to policing and other first responder communities.

So, how is it that this tribe is formed? At the core of the answer to that question is a concept known as *Social Identity Theory*.

Our social identity is the part of one's self-concept that comes from affiliation with different social groups. A couple of the bigwigs who developed this concept throughout the 1970s and 80s are social psychologists Henri Tajfel and John Turner.

Tajfel and Turner propose that a big chunk of our identities is related to the groups that we are a part of, which are referred to as our *in-groups*. By this definition, groups that we are not a part of become *out-groups* and certain intergroup behaviours can be predicted based on perception of group status differences.

When you start to look for social identity theory at play, you can see it everywhere. One obvious place is fans of sporting teams. Those who barrack for one team will perceive their in-group of followers as superior to those out-groups who barrack for other teams (often despite any tangible evidence from the scoreboard to validate that perceived superiority!)

For the most part this in-group affiliation is relatively innocent. Although it can occasionally escalate to violence, generally, it is nothing more than a bit of innocent heckling of out-groups and the odd derogatory comment, which serves to help strengthen in-group cohesiveness at the expense of members of the out-group.

Stepping up from that basic example, we see social identity theory playing out with cultural and racial divides and history is littered with disastrous examples of those divides being taken to extremes.

Bringing the discussion back to the military and first responder communities, the start of in-group identity formation begins at the point of selection for the role. What happens there is a distillation of society to some degree, with those selected for roles such as policing, firefighting, paramedicine, and military service, being taken from let's say the upper 50% of society with respect to overall physical and intellectual functioning. Those with significant physical or mental health issues are excluded, as are those with criminal histories, or those who might fail any basic security screening process required for acceptance into the organisation.

Due to the nature of the process, it's easy to lose sight of the fact that this has occurred. A new Bell Curve is formed over the trainee or recruit cohort and a pecking order of performance is established with high and low performers identified. What gets lost in this redistribution is the acknowledgement that even perceived *low performers* within the new in-group are relatively high performing when compared to the broader population they were selected from.

Induction into the training pipeline for the new role is often a particularly significant departure from the individual's previous social identity and is marked by ceremonies such as issuing of uniforms and potentially strict regulations around shaving, hair length and styles, piercings, etc. These factors all serve to reinforce a sense of membership to the organisational in-group. In doing so, they also strengthen the divide between the cohort and what is now the out-group of broader society.

In the military setting, this becomes a divide between the military in-group and the civilian out-group. Military identity is often strengthened by the ignorant perspective that civilians are somehow a lesser species, who are undisciplined and always running late for things! While this is a great way to build moral and a sense of esprit de corps within a military in-group, you can begin to see how it can be quite toxic at the end of a career when a transitioning military member once again finds themselves suddenly thrust back into civilian life, having spent their career seeing *civvies* as an out-group. It is literally the exact opposite of their social identity to be a civilian.

As a military member or first responder progresses through their training pipeline their in-group affiliation is strengthened through shared hardship with fellow recruits or trainees. Key milestones, such as graduation or qualification, are marked with specific ceremonies that serve to indoctrinate the new group into the broader tribe of the organisation. From there, experience in the role further strengthens social identity with the in-group and distance from out-groups.

A member might further progress within their organisation to specialist roles such as police negotiators, police tactical groups, corrections emergency response groups, military special operations, or intensive care qualifications as a paramedic. In these instances, another distillation of the in-group, and shifting of the Bell Curve occurs, and a refined in-group identity is developed.

For me, this process evolved through entry into the military (making civilians an out-group) and furthermore my choice to join the army, making Air Force and Navy out-groups as well (despite them being part of my broader military in-group). From there I held several unit in-group identities before moving into special operations. At that stage, the special operations in-group made the broader army an out-group and the concept of being a civilian was a distant memory. This process is graphically represented in Figure 1.

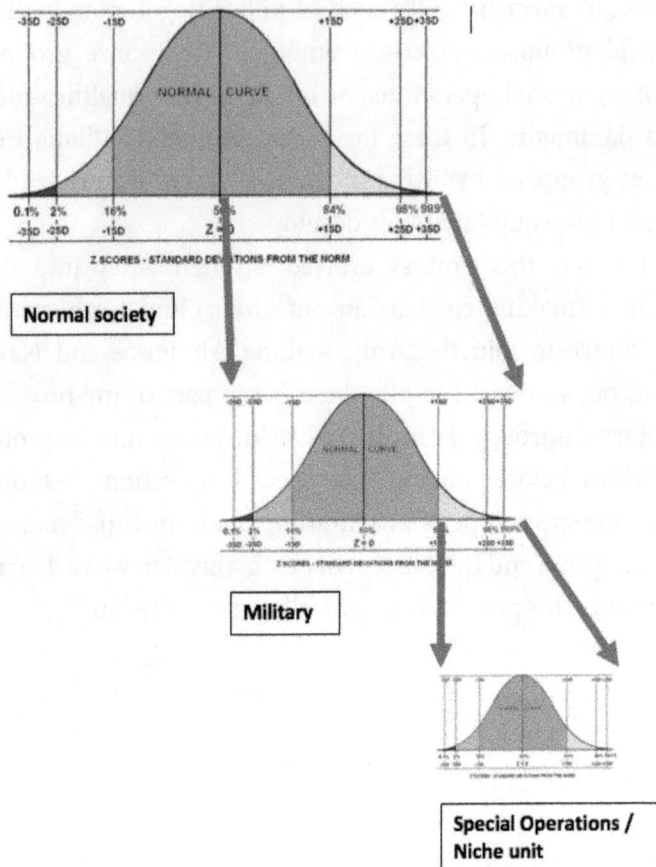

Figure 1. The distillation of society on entry into the military, and then furthermore on acceptance into special operations.

As most will experience as they progress in their organisation, I had increasingly intense experiences, both positive and negative, and the sharing of these experiences with members of my tribe strengthened our joint social identity. At the same time, it distanced us further from out-groups including not only civilians but the broader military who weren't routinely being utilised in the same capacity as special operations and thus weren't having the same experiences to be able to relate to. Over time in this sort of environment the next level of group cohesion often occurs, known as *identity fusion*.

Identity Fusion

Identity fusion is described as having a *visceral sense of oneness* with a group. Individual identity has overlapped with group identity and a kin-like relationship is formed (or perceived) with other group members.

Returning to the social identity theory example of sporting team fans used above, it's likely that if fellow fans of a sporting team met in a bar that they would have a chat and perhaps have a beer together, but it's less likely that they would lay down their life for one another if things went loud (with the obvious exception of hardcore soccer fans!)

On the other hand, the identity fused individual probably would risk their own personal safety for other tribe members, even if they don't know the other member particularly well, or even if they don't particularly like them as a person. The fact that they are a member of the tribal in-group that their identity is fused with dictates that they will help.

Think of a firefighter turning up to a burning building and knowing that a firefighter from a different team is in there, or the police officer being called to the scene of an active shooter knowing that cops from a different jurisdiction are in the hot zone. In both instances, I would bet that the backup team wouldn't hesitate to risk their own lives to help. You could argue that they would both also act if it were anyone trapped in the building or hot zone, however the urge to act is likely to be more intense if it's one of their own tribe members at risk.

Although this process of identity fusion is fantastic at bonding the tribe into a tight knit entity, the added level of investment serves to psychologically draw the individual away from their affiliation with other groups they may have formerly been, or still are, a member of. It is possible to be identity fused with multiple groups, but it's difficult due to the requirement for investment of time and energy into those groups to remain at that level of membership.

An obvious struggle here is the military member or first responder who has a family. Becoming identity fused with a work tribe creates pressures that not only physically take the individual away from their family to meet the time commitments of operational requirements with their work tribe, but also creates a psychological distance from the family tribe. This is due to the unique exposures of the work role (or perhaps security considerations) that distance the member from their family who, through absolutely no fault of their own, cannot begin to associate with (or aren't given the opportunity to know about in the security setting).

After a while it just becomes easier to go all-in with the work tribe and loosen ties with other group affiliations.

Once this occurs, the identity fused individual has often let go of their non-family relationships that existed before they became indoctrinated into their tribe, and relationships with family can become strained and distanced. Maintaining membership with wider groups such as sporting teams or other hobby groups outside of work or family becomes an almost impossible proposition.

While everything is going well in the professional life of the identity fused individual then things are rosy. They will often be growing and progressing professionally and further establishing themselves within their tribe. As time passes, newer members will join the tribe and look to them as leaders and mentors, bolstering their status and sense of personal significance and purpose (key factors contributing to a positive individual identity). All continues to go well right up until the time comes to transition out of the tribe.

Understanding the process described in this chapter of forming a social identity and then progressing to identity fusion as a military member or first responder allows us to appreciate the psychological impact of transition.

When I consider my own experience, in the grand scheme of things I had spent a relatively short period of time in the military (a little under 15 years) but in that time I had invested deeply in my work identity. I had completely shed my civilian identity and fallen headfirst into the trap of looking down my nose at civvies. I had been indoctrinated into the army social identity group and then progressed to identity fusion in my role as a doctor with army special operations. I had completely disengaged from any civilian groups that I had previously been a member of, and I was distanced from my immediate family group due to the time spent away from them during my service, compounded by the security requirements of the job and the foreign nature of my exposures that were unrelatable to my immediate family.

The second that I took my army uniform off for the last time and discharged, I was cast out from the military in-group and (by definition at least) became a civilian again. I was now, once again, a member of the very group that I had considered an out-group for the previous 15-odd years and who I had ignorantly convinced myself were inferior. Yet there I was as a civilian again. I didn't want to be one of them and what's more, I couldn't remember how to be one. I hadn't kept any ties with any civilian groups that might have better facilitated reintegration and I didn't have any hobbies or interests in civilian life to potentially reintegrate to those in-groups.

I still identified as military and my identity was still fused with my special operations tribe, but I was no longer part of either of those in-groups.

From an evolutionary perspective, being dislocated from one's tribe was a disastrous outcome that often meant a very real threat to life. The safety from predators that the tribe offered was lost, as was the access to the collective group hunting and gathering efforts to provide food and resources for all to survive. The lone individual was at very real risk of death. While the risk of death from exposure or starvation no longer exists to anywhere near the same degree as it did in ancient civilisations, the stress response of isolation from tribe is still activated within us as it was back in the day, causing anxiety, depression, and a deep sense of loneliness.

When we consider a normal healthy identity, it should be influenced by a variety of different groups. Let's look at a typical adolescent who is going through the process of resolving their identity crisis and working towards identity achievement. They'll be a member of a family, whatever that looks like to them, will likely have a social circle of friends, and let's say they're a member of a social group or two, and play some social sport. As they enter further studies, training for a trade, or perhaps the workforce, their identity could be depicted as illustrated in Figure 2, with a healthy amount of influence from all groups.

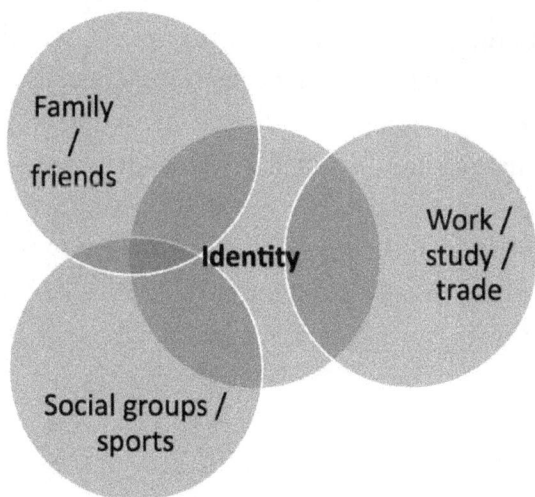

Figure 2. A balanced identity influenced by a variety of social groups in healthy amounts.

At the risk of generalisation, it is assumed that the role they're assuming in further studies, trade training, or the workforce, is less likely than a military or first responder role to lead to an all-consuming sense of social identity or the potential for identity fusion.

As the individual starts to form their adult identity it is balanced out by a healthy range of social identities. They will feel affiliated with their role, but not to the point of exclusion of group membership in their family, friend, social, and sporting groups. They generally aren't isolated from these other groups and thrust into the unique environment that the military member or first responder finds themselves when entering academies or training pipelines and their exposures and experiences are more relatable to the wider population, which makes association and understanding easier. As a result, they stay psychologically better connected with the general population during the formation of their adult identity.

For the reasons discussed above, if that same individual enters the military or a first responder role, they are likely to commence on the pathway towards identity fusion and their ties with family and links to other societal groups are strained or broken. Diagrammatically, they look more like Figure 3.

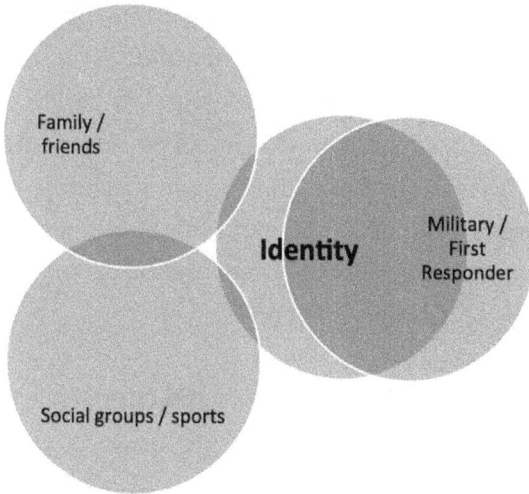

Figure 3. Identity fusion with a military or first responder tribe causing distancing from family, friends and other social or sporting groups.

The loss of this hard-earned social identity can be confronting during transition; however, being aware of it is part of identifying the psychology at play to help formulate a roadmap out of the darkness.

Remember the sage words of Matty McConaughey:

"Once you know it's black, it's not near as dark"

If you've transitioned out of the military or a first responder role, it's probable that you still feel socially attached and perhaps identity fused with your former tribal group, but it's essential to face the fact that you are no longer part of that in-group.

Just as it took years to decades to form the tribal affiliation with your work group, you can expect it to take years to form the same level of bond with a new group, but the first step is acceptance of transition out of the former tribe. This doesn't mean you need to cut ties with members of that former tribe (more on that in chapters to come) but it does mean you need to be proactive in engaging with new social groups to productively move forward in life and work towards new identity achievement and not get stuck in the black space of identity diffusion.

Call to action: What is your social identity?

Complete the following diagram by drawing a solid line in place of the dotted one in the position you feel it currently overlaps with the various social groups.

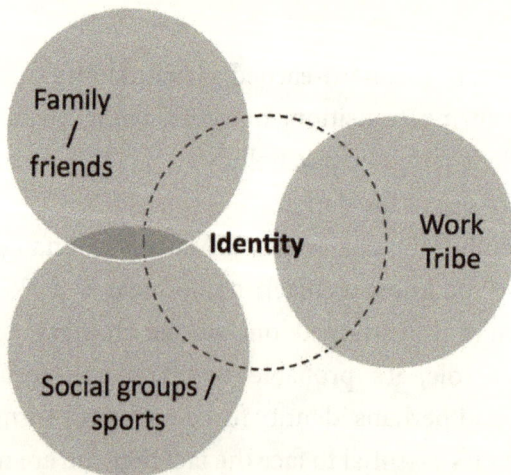

Consider the following questions:

1. Could you invest more in your social identity as a family member or friend?

2. Are there friendships outside of work you've let go that you'd like to pick back up?

3. Are there social or sporting groups that you've either let go due to work commitments, or might be interested in joining post-transition?

4. If you have a new role post-transition, are you underinvested in that identity? If so, how could you invest more in your new work identity?

5. If you break it, you buy it!

When I was a kid, I recall seeing signs in lots of shops that stated *if you break it; you buy it*. The meaning was unambiguous to me, and I knew that if I were to handle something in the shop and drop it or damage it in any way then I would be expected to pay for it.

To this day, the concept makes perfect sense to me although I don't seem to see those signs around as much any longer. For the same reason that it seems reasonable to me that I should pay for something in a store that I might have broken while playing with it, it seems reasonable to me that an organisation should pay for members who become broken during their service.

For the most part, contingency exists for this to occur, although I certainly appreciate that individual experiences with these systems vary dramatically and not everyone has a positive outcome. At the time of writing this book I am yet to put in any claims for service-related issues and embarrassingly, it took me nine years after my discharge to even register as a veteran with the Australian Department of Veterans Affairs.

There were multiple reasons for this significant delay. Firstly, I'm slack! Plain, and simple! Secondly, I was very lucky not to suffer any career ending physical or mental health injuries from my service that would have necessitated an earlier registration. But thirdly, another couple of key barriers to my lodging any service-related claims are a personal unease with the term *entitlement*, as well as a reluctance to accept any form of *disability identity*, no matter how relatively small it might be compared to others.

I have discussed these third lot of reasons with many military and first responder members who have transitioned and who share this mindset. It makes sense, it's the very mindset that made them so effective in the role. They went in as volunteers, they deliberately made the bed that they ended up lying in, and if they copped a few bangs and scratches along the way then they take ownership for that.

I also hear that the reluctance of some to seek any form of compensation is seeded in the deep desire to avoid being associated with others who have adopted a strong *disability identity*. This is particularly prevalent with mental health diagnoses and often the desire to not be stamped with a PTSD diagnosis. I get it, I was one of those discharging veterans. This mindset then results in the transitioning member not seeking any support, rehabilitation, or compensation at all for their service-related issues and can lead to a certain degree of resentment to the organisation they have transitioned out of, not to mention sub-optimal management of their conditions.

At the extreme other end of this spectrum exists those who have become identity fused with the disability identity and perhaps even (mostly unconsciously) adopted a victim mentality. In this extreme, the individual might start to feel that they have no control over their own future and that they are outsourcing their wellbeing to their former organisation to fund, and their treating medical and psychological team to facilitate. I'm not for one second suggesting that the individual wants this outcome or has deliberately chosen it. I fear that in some instances the system can drive the circumstances in this direction.

From my vantage point, this is what has happened to several of my former friends and colleagues. One case study that comes to mind was a former army special operations soldier and friend of mine who I'll call Scotty (not his real name). Scotty was well established in his unit and had completed multiple operational tours of war zones. Over his time, he had accumulated several niggling physical injuries and, on what would end up being his final operation tour, he was involved in an incident that weighed heavily on him from a psychological perspective. On return from that tour his physical injuries were starting to limit his ability to perform his role, so he underwent surgery to try to fix them. During his physical rehabilitation period his mental health started to deteriorate due to rumination on the incident he was involved in.

After a period of psychological management, he was eventually referred to a psychiatrist and a formal diagnosis of PTSD was made, rendering Scotty unsuitable for service in his role as a special operator while he had ongoing psychiatric treatment.

He continued to turn up to work but couldn't perform his former role and hence was given other more menial tasks to fill his time. This put him on the outer of his tribe of special operators (the perceived *lower end* of the special operations Bell Curve) and a distance began to form between him and his tribe. Scotty's sense of significance and purpose deteriorated, and his mental health worsened. Unfortunately, his surgery had not been successful in fixing his physical injuries and things started to head in the direction of a medical discharge from the army, causing further deterioration in Scotty's mental health.

As he worsened, his treating psychiatrist recommended that he not attend the workplace at all due to concerns that it served as a trigger to his previous traumatic experiences. As the process of his medical discharge progressed, Scotty began to adopt a disability identity in place of his former identity as a highly functioning special operations soldier. His new fight became that of convincing the system that he was indeed broken, to secure a pension and his financial security on discharge. As should be the case, the more broken he could demonstrate he was from his service, the higher his pension would be. Scotty's claims were 100% legitimate, but I watched with dismay as he was required repeatedly to state his claims of disability and fight the system to acknowledge that he had become *totally and permanently incapacitated* due to his service. I can only imagine what that label alone would have done for Scotty's mental health!

With so much of the process existing completely outside of Scotty's ability to control or influence, it made sense to me that he was forced into a degree of victim mentality during the process. He quite literally was along for the ride when it came to his professional and financial future being determined by the powers to be. Eventually he was discharged on a pension and despite gallant efforts to rebuild himself, Scotty lost his ongoing battle and became yet another veteran statistic.

Now I appreciate that there were many factors going on in Scotty's life that I had no idea about and I'm not for one moment suggesting that he consciously adopted a victim mentality. Furthermore, I'm not passing judgement on what happened here, or in any other similar case, I'm simply making observations from my perspective. A former highly functioning special operations soldier was physically and mentally injured and despite everyone's best efforts and intentions, he ended up losing his sense of significance and purpose, losing his job, losing his tribe, being cast out of his in-group, labelled by the system as totally and permanently incapacitated, and ultimately losing his life.

Locus of Control

When it comes to the adoption or avoidance of a victim mentality, a key concept to understand is *locus of control*.

American psychologist Julian Rotter developed the

concept of locus of control in the 1950s and it basically describes the amount we feel we can influence the outcome of any given situation.

Locus of control exists on a spectrum from the negative end (*external locus of control*), where we feel disempowered and like we have no ability to influence what happens in our lives, to the positive end (*internal locus of control*), where we feel like we're in the driver's seat of our lives and can influence the outcome of situations directly.

Locus of Control

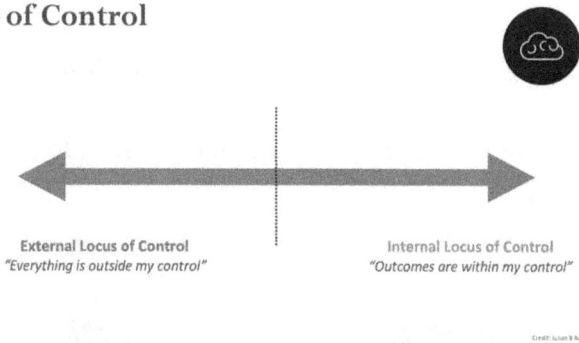

External Locus of Control
"Everything is outside my control"

Internal Locus of Control
"Outcomes are within my control"

Credit: Julian B Rotter

Figure 4. Rotter's Locus of Control spectrum (Image source: The Resilience Shield course content)

This is not new wisdom, with Stoic philosophy from two thousand years ago being littered with references to the concept. Here are a couple of my favourites:

"You have power over your mind, not outside events. Realize this, and you will find strength". Marcus Aurelius

"Happiness and freedom begin with a clear understanding of one principle; Some things are within
our control and some things are not". Epictetus

Whenever possible, we want to drive our locus of
control towards the internal end of the spectrum but to do
this we need a realistic appreciation of what we can and
can't control or influence.

Building on Rotter's work is Steven Covey (author of the
book *7 Habits of Highly Effective People*) who distinguishes
between *proactive* people, who focus on what they can do
and influence, and reactive people, who focus their energy
on things beyond their control and are prone to a victim
mentality.

Covey uses a model based on two circles to illustrate his
concept.

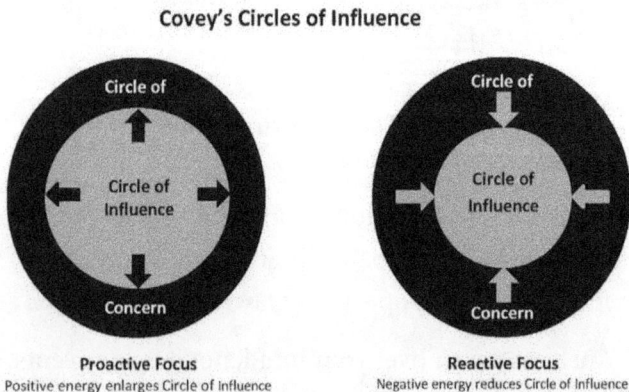

Covey's Circles of Influence

Circle of

Circle of
Influence

Concern

Proactive Focus
Positive energy enlarges Circle of Influence

Circle of

Circle of
Influence

Concern

Reactive Focus
Negative energy reduces Circle of Influence

Figure 5. Covey's Circles of Influence (Image source: https://dplearn-
ingzone.the-dp.co.uk)

Covey's model is based on two circles. The outer *Circle of Concern* describes all the factors in our lives that concern us but that we don't have any ability to control or influence. The inner *Circle of Influence* is the stuff that we can either directly control or, at least, realistically have an influence on.

To drive our locus of control towards the internal end of the spectrum, the goal is to identify what situations in our lives exist in what circles and then focus our energy only on the things in our circle of influence. It's easier said than done, but we need to try to let go of the things in our circle of concern because no amount of emotional energy spent in this space is going to influence the outcome. Furthermore, the more energy wasted in our circle of concern, the further we reinforce an external locus of control (the perception we can't influence things) and risk adopting a victim mentality.

Let's have a look at how this applies to the transitioning member who has accumulated some service-related injuries over the years. In my opinion (only now, nearly a decade after discharge!) it makes perfect sense to put in claims for any legitimate injuries relating to service. This requires overcoming the mentality of being someone who doesn't ask for help, and the mindset that ffears association with a disability identity. Approach it from the perspective of the *you broke it; you buy it* philosophy.

With that said, the next step is to apply Covey's circle model to the situation. The transitioning member can directly influence their attendance at medical and psychological appointments for review and accurate diagnosis of service-related conditions, however they need to appreciate that the ultimate outcome of any claims exists in their *circle of concern*.

Once the claim is lodged, the best thing they can be doing is then focusing their physical and emotional energy on rehabilitation and trying not to invest energy in the outcome of claims process (once again, I get it; easier said than done).

If a diagnosis is established, then by definition the member has a disability identity thrust upon them, but this needn't be a negative thing. With a degree of *cognitive reframing*, the positives of the situation might be seen. For example, participation in initiatives such as the Invictus Games for wounded servicemen and women (or equivalent for other services) might become a focus for transitioning military members to positively reframe their disability identity. Likewise, if appropriate, becoming an advocate of mentor for other injured transitioning military members or first responders might be another positive way to embrace a disability identity. Whatever works for the individual, but it's the focus on the *ability* component that counts.

Remember, our identities are made up of the individual factors outlined in Chapter 3, as well our social identities relating to the in-groups we are a part of (Chapter 4). One risk for the member transitioning due to medical or psychological injury is that they adopt a victim mentality and become identity fused with their disability identity. This risk must be fought with every resource the member has, focusing on their circle of influence, with every attempt made to let go of things in their circle of concern, and a balanced investment in parts of their identity other than their disability identity.

To round out this chapter, I'd like to use another one of my favourite Stoic quotes from the great Marcus Aurelius:

"Get busy with life's purpose, toss aside empty hopes, get active in your own rescue – if you care for yourself at all – and do it while you can".

Call to action: Assess your Locus of Control

Do you have an internal (positive) or external (negative) locus of control?

There are several scales that can be used to give you an insight into where your locus of control lies. An internet search will reveal a few that you can do for free online. I recommend starting with Rotter's Locus of Control Scale and go from there. Remember to answer the questions honestly and not how you feel will give you the best-looking results. If you do identify that you have an external locus of control, then use the ancient Stoic wisdom and Covey's Circle Model to turn your focus on your circle of influence (things you can control or influence) and away from your circle of concern (things outside of your ability to control or influence).

Have you legitimately been injured by your service?

This isn't about taking the piss and fabricating or embellishing injuries from your military or first responder careers, it's about breaking down the counterproductive mindset of not claiming for legitimate injuries from your service and doing the things you can control or influence to have these injuries recognised.

Getting active in your own rescue here involves being proactive in accessing your service medical and psychological files, seeking the appropriate assistance in lodging claims, and then attending appointments to assess and validate your injury status. The focus should be on positively developing and following rehabilitation plans to get back to the best physical and mental version of yourself you can be following transition. Remember, the ultimate outcome of your claims exists outside of your control (in your circle of concern), so try to let that go and focus on what you can control and influence instead.

Sometimes, service-related injuries may not be as obvious as you might think. The compounding effect of many varied exposures over a career in the military or a first responder role can cause insidious injuries that are not immediately attributable to one specific incident.

It is recognised that military and first responder roles cause significantly higher cumulative physical and mental stress on the individual than more *normal* jobs, which is referred to as *allostatic load*. Recent research in this area by

Frueh et al (2020)[8] has led to the term *Operator Syndrome* to encompass the:

> "...natural consequences of an extraordinarily high allostatic load; the accumulation of physiological, neural, and neuroendocrine responses resulting from the prolonged chronic stress; and physical demands of a career with the military special forces".

While this article focuses in on the somewhat extreme exposures of military special forces soldiers, the same pattern of health issues can be seen to varying degrees across the full range of military and first response roles. I highly recommend that anyone reading this book should also read Frueh et al's article (you can find the reference in the footnotes) to further understand some of the less obvious physical and mental health consequences of their service and perhaps to guide their claims process.

A sense of purpose and motivation are the topics of the next chapter, so set yourself the purpose of optimising your physical and mental health in transition and get motivated towards those goals!

---

8 Frueh BC, Madan A, Fowler JC, Stomberg S, Bradshaw M, Kelly K, Weinstein B, Luttrell M, Danner SG, Beidel DC. "Operator syndrome": A unique constellation of medical and behavioral health-care needs of military special operation forces. Int J Psychiatry Med. 2020 Jul;55(4):281-295.

6. You will lose your sense of purpose and motivation

Our sense of purpose and what motivates us to do what we do are other things that most of us inherently know, but few of us take the time to define in any great detail. Both purpose and motivation can generally be found in abundance within military or first response organisations. During the training pipeline for these roles the motivation is to achieve the required standard to progress towards qualification and graduation. The sense of purpose is strengthened along the way. Be that to serve your country in a military capacity, or serve your community as a police officer, firefighter, intelligence officer, paramedic, or correctional officer, the purpose is one of contributing to something bigger than yourself, answering calls for help from the community, and perhaps even making the difference between life and death.

This sense of purpose is reflected in the mottos of such organisations, including the LAPD's *To Protect and To Serve* and *That Others May Live* in the instance of the US Air Forces' Pararescuemen.

As with all the psychological concepts discussed throughout this book, there are many models of human motivation. The one that I find most relevant to the military and first responder communities, is Maslow's Hierarchy of Needs.

As the name suggests, Maslow's hierarchy of needs is exactly that, a hierarchical list of human needs that, if all are met, can ultimately result in what Maslow termed *self-actualisation* (Maslow, 1943)[9]. Maslow's Hierarchy is often represented diagrammatically as a pyramid (see Figure 6), with its foundation being the basic physiological needs such as air, water, food, shelter, clothing, sleep etc.

Once those basic needs are met, the considerations that form the next block of the pyramid are the safety needs and include personal safety and security, health, employment, and other fundamental resources. These first two building blocks that form the base of the pyramid are considered the *basic needs* of a human and Maslow considered them to be the primary motivators for human behaviour. While it's not impossible to progress upward in Maslow's Hierarchy without the basic needs being met (during his incarceration, Nelson Mandela is a great example of someone who did) it certainly is difficult.

Once the basic needs are fulfilled, which is the case for most living in contemporary developed-world societies, the next levels of the pyramid are belongingness and love

---

[9] Maslow, A. H. (1943). A theory of human motivation. *Psychological Review*, 50(4), 370–396.

needs, which are met through relationships with intimate partners and friends. Once these are established, Maslow proposed that the individual will be motivated by esteem needs, being the desire for prestige and feelings of accomplishment. Coupled together, the belongingness, love, and esteem needs, are referred to as the *psychological needs* of an individual, and if met can lead to fulfilment in those who don't crave more out of life.

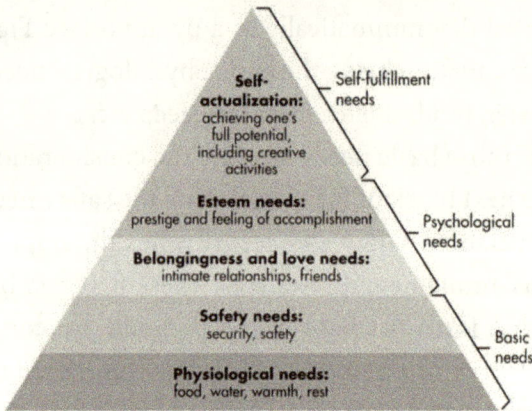

Figure 6. Maslow's Hierarchy of Needs
(Image source: www.simplypsychology.org)

Maslow hypothesised that for most people however, even if all the basic and psychological needs are satisfied, that a new restlessness will develop unless they are doing what they are best fitted to do. Maslow referred to this as the need for *self-actualisation*, which is characterised by becoming the best version of oneself and reaching ones' full potential. Maslow suggested that self-actualisers are typically creative, autonomous, objective individuals who are concerned about humanity and accepting of themselves and others[10].

Maslow's theory of self-actualisation falls into the category of what are known as eudemonic philosophies, which can be traced back to Aristotle's (384-322 BC) notion of eudemonia or being true to one's inner demon. Common among these philosophies is the premise that people should develop what's best within themselves and then use those skills and talents for a greater good, particularly the welfare of other people or mankind as a whole[11].

Military, law enforcement, fire services, ambulance and other first response services are all organisations that promote individual excellence and exist to a large degree for the greater good of society. It therefore figures that many individuals who enter military or first responder roles are those who crave self-actualisation as defined by Maslow.

Once indoctrinated into a military or first response organisation and established in a specific role, a well-defined pathway to progress upwards in Maslow's Hierarchy exists. The member is likely to be earning sufficient money to provide for their basic needs and that of their family, and they usually have a decent degree of job security. Belongingness and esteem needs can be met by the professional

---

[10] Maslow, A. H. (1943). A theory of human motivation. *Psychological Review*, 50(4), 370–396.

[11] Peterson, C., Park, N. & Seligman, M.E.P. Orientations to happiness and life satisfaction: the full life versus the empty life. *J Happiness Stud* 6, 25–41 (2005).

satisfaction and respect earned from being a highly functioning team member, and the process of training and indoctrination into the organisation will facilitate the tribal sense of affiliation discussed in Chapter 4, helping to fulfil the psychological requirements of Maslow's Hierarchy.

Whether or not the individual has intimate relationships outside of their work environment, it is still likely that a significant degree of their close friends will come from other members of their organisation.

Throughout a well-structured military or first responder career, a member will undergo ongoing professional development courses to learn new skills, challenge themselves, and experience the accomplishment of progressing up the ranks, fulfilling their esteem needs as they do so. The opportunity to self-actualise by *being all they can be* in their work role is then available to them through using their skills in contribution towards a greater good and the service of others.

With hindsight, I can see clearly that I was self-actualised in my role as a doctor with army special operations. I was earning plenty of money to provide for my own basic needs and that of my family, I had a tribal sense of belongingness with my work colleagues and a sense of prestige and accomplishment that came from using my skills in complex environments, regularly in life-or-death situations. I honestly felt that I was the very best version of myself and was doing what I had been put on the planet to do. In Maslow's terms, I was self-actualised.

There was just one catch that I hadn't completely registered at the time. My self-actualisation was *as a doctor with army special operations* and not as an individual outside of that role. The second I took my uniform off I lost my sense of self-actualisation, my feelings of prestige and esteem, my sense of accomplishment, and a large chunk of my feelings of belongingness that had come from being part of that tribal in-group. Thankfully, my relationship with my wife and young family had stayed intact, allowing me to maintain a percentage of my psychological needs, but the rest was stripped away immediately upon my transition out of my military role. I had failed to realise the following truth:

Most of the prestige belongs to the uniform and not to you.

Diagrammatically, what had occurred looked something like Figure 7.

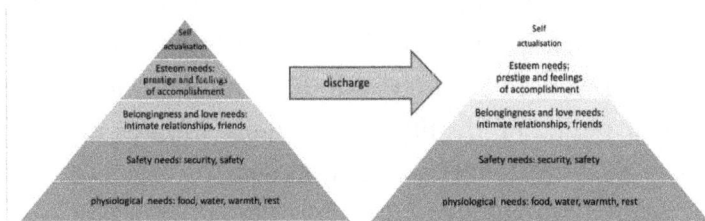

Figure 7. The loss of self-actualisation, prestige and esteem, and work-related belongingness and friends following discharge.

I had been identity fused with my military role and the loss of that identity left me not really knowing who I was out of uniform. As previously mentioned, I had also spent

15-odd years bolstering my military in-group identity by thinking less of the civilian out-group, and in the blink of an eye I had become a civilian again.

As unsettling as all of this was for years post-transition, realising what had occurred through the lens of Maslow's model was hugely instructive in rebuilding myself. It wasn't easy, in fact it was tremendously difficult, however the principles were simple. I needed to rebuild the upper layers of my Maslow's Hierarchy in new life domains. I needed to find a new tribe and seek esteem, prestige, and feelings of accomplishment elsewhere. I realised that it was only through doing this that I was ever going to experience self-actualisation again.

Just as it took me years to reach the point of self-actu-alisation in my military role, I could expect it to take years to reach that point again in a new life endeavour. Just as I had tried on multiple identities in my initial adolescent period of identity crisis before I accomplished my military identity, I would need to try out different things to resolve my new period of identity crisis to move towards my new post-transition identity accomplishment.

Ikigai

Another model that I have found useful to this discussion is the Japanese construct known as *ikigai*[12]. The term comes

---

[12] To read further on the concept of ikigai, check out Garcia, H. & Miralles, F. 2017, Ikigai: The Japanese secret to a long and happy life, Huthinson Publishing Trade.

from an amalgam of "iki", meaning *alive* or *life*, and "gai", meaning *benefit* or *worth*. Combined, ikigai roughly refers to what gives our life worth, meaning, and purpose. Ikigai exists at the intersection of the following four things:

- What you love
- What the world needs
- What you can be paid for
- What you are good at

Ikigai is diagrammatically represented as Figure 8.

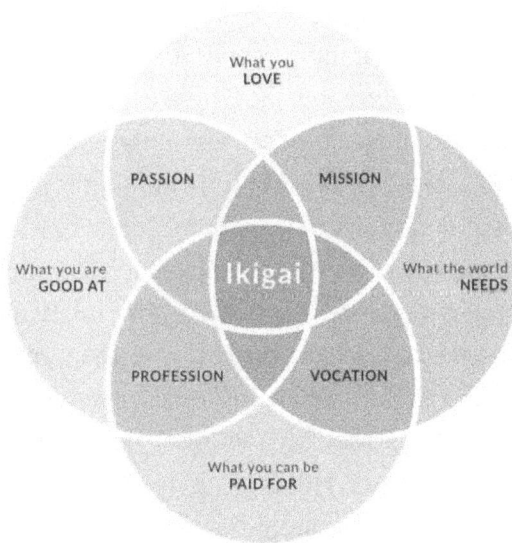

Figure 8. Ikigai exists at the intersection of what you love, what the world needs, what you can get paid for, and what you're good at. (Image source: www.forbes.com)

There are many parallels between ikigai and Maslow's concept of self-actualisation. Once again, reflecting on my time as a doctor with army special operations, I consider that I had found my ikigai at the time.

Many military members and first responders will be able to associate with the feeling of ikigai from some point in their career. Often it first occurs throughout the training pipeline and then continues well into their operational role with their organisation. During that period, they often have a love for the role, have become good at it, can clearly see the need for their skills in the world, and are taking home a paycheck every fortnight.

Considering ikigai more deeply, it becomes evident that the four components that make it up are transient, therefore the experience of ikigai itself can also only ever be transient.

What you love changes over time, sometimes in military and first responder roles the love of the job can be lost as cumulative exposures or career pressures increase. Individuals may no longer be as good at the role as they might once have been, perhaps due to physical injuries or the normal aging process taking its toll. What the world needs might shift with societal changes and technological developments such as artificial intelligence, which might lead to certain aspects of roles, or certain roles completely, becoming obsolete and therefore no longer something that pay a wage.

If you are one of the lucky ones who found and maintained ikigai in your work role throughout your career leading up to transition, then that is fantastic. But you must then appreciate that ikigai will be lost in transition (parallel to the stripping of the top layers of Maslow's Hierarchy).

If you're like many military members and first responders, you may have found that either you never really hit a point of ikigai in your role, or more likely, you were once there but over time had fallen out of love with the role. This will have left you somewhere between the *vocation* and *profession* sections of the ikigai model. The world still needed what you were doing, you could still get paid for it, and you were good at it, you just didn't love it any longer.

Whether you found and kept ikigai throughout your career, found it then lost it, or never found it at all, the fact remains that post-transition you're going to need to recreate some (and hopefully all) of the components of it. What you need to focus on depends on what stage in life you're at when you transition.

Transition prior to retirement age

If you're transitioning prior to retirement age, then you will most likely need to find something new you can get paid for. Ideally that will be something that you love, but a good place to start searching is on the list of your professional qualifications and skills (what you're good at) that you created in Chapter 3. Map this against what the world needs and you're starting to hone in on a new professional role. Remember to also consider your values in this equation and ideally search for roles that are aligned with your personal values.

If you can find a new role that you happen to love then great, you just might be able to achieve a new state of ikigai. In the absence of that, the *passion* and *mission* areas of the ikigai diagram can provide guidance as to other things you can use to recreate a fulfilling life post-transition.

If your new work is more of a vocation or profession that's fine, you can balance that out with things outside of work that you love and the world needs (missions) and things you love and that you're good at (passions) to create a *composite ikigai*.

A lot of transitioning military and first response members are looking to recapture the stimulus and satisfaction of their former role in their next job, but that often isn't achievable. You don't need to get everything from your work role, as long as you're accomplishing all four of the key aspects of ikigai in some area of your life, you're on the right track to progressing back up Maslow's Hierarchy.

Transition at retirement age

All going to plan, there will be less emphasis on the requirement to find something you can get paid for if you're transitioning at retirement age. That said, part time work can be a very fulfilling aspect of life in retirement, as can missions such as unpaid work as a volunteer. Perhaps you can use some of the unique skills you have acquired during your working life to contribute towards training or mentoring the next generation coming through in your former profession. Doing so can provide a fantastic sense of self-worth and esteem and help to rebuild the psychological layers of your Maslow's Hierarchy that were lost on retirement.

Likewise, it's important to find passions in your life. While the ikigai construct suggests that a passion exists at the intersection of what you love and what you're good at, I would argue that you don't need to particularly good at something to be passionate about it. You just need to be good enough. Joining hobby or sporting groups can be a great way to develop and express passions, make new friends, contribute to a sense of belongingness, and accomplishment as you improve your skills. Who knows, you might even find yourself a new tribe!

Transition due to medical or psychological reasons

This is likely to be the toughest scenario of all, especially if you have been forced out of a role that you had found ikigai and self-actualisation in. I'm the first to admit that I cannot personally empathise with this situation as I haven't lived it. That said, I believe that the models of Maslow's Hierarchy and ikigai are instructive in how to best rebuild yourself under these circumstances.

It may be that you need to start rebuilding your Maslow's Hierarchy from the very bottom. Hopefully, your old organisation has taken some responsibility for your physical or psychological situation, and you're in receipt of some form of pension in acknowledgement of your service-related injuries. If this isn't the case, then you need to do your very best to avoid slipping into a victim mentality and an external locus of control. Remember the Stoic wisdom from the previous chapter and focus your emotional energy on what you can control and influence. Use the attributes that made you the highly functioning member of your previous tribe and claw your way back to meeting your basic needs in whatever way is possible. Once there, or in the instance that you are in receipt of a pension that allows you to financially meet your basic needs, it is critical to then pursue the higher levels of Maslow's Hierarchy once more.

I'm of the firm belief that *you cannot buy self-esteem*.

In Maslow's Hierarchy, money only really allows you to fulfil your basic needs, and in ikigai it only contributes to one-quarter of the factors that give our life worth, meaning, and purpose. We need to actively seek out the others. Even if you are physically or psychologically limited by service-related injuries, you must seek out new friends and ideally a sense of tribe, and new avenues to feel accomplishment and prestige. Looking again at ikigai, these can be found in passions and missions. Even if you are in receipt of a full pension that might disincentivise or disallow paid work, and as difficult as it may be, you still need to strive for these things.

Call to action: What factors are making up your Maslow's Hierarchy?

First, consider the factors that contributed to the various layers of your Maslow's Hierarchy prior to transition by completing the following diagram.

Were you self-actualised? If so, what made you feel that way?

Self-Actualisation

Where did you get your sense of esteem, prestige, and accomplishment?

Esteem and Prestige Needs

Where did your sense of belongingness come from?

Belongingness Needs

How were you meeting your basic needs?

Basic Needs

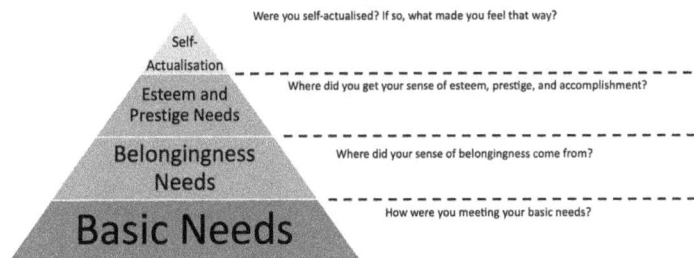

Next, consider what your Maslow's Hierarchy might look like post-transition by completing the following diagram.

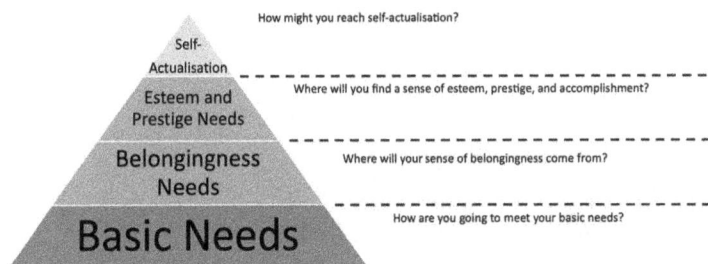

How might you reach self-actualisation?

Self-Actualisation

Where will you find a sense of esteem, prestige, and accomplishment?

Esteem and Prestige Needs

Where will your sense of belongingness come from?

Belongingness Needs

How are you going to meet your basic needs?

Basic Needs

Call to Action: Finding (or re-finding) post-transition ikigai

Complete the following table listing the components of ikigai (use your list of professional qualifications and skills from Chapter 3 as a starting point for what you're good at):

What do you love?	What does the world need that you can contribute to?
What can you get paid for?	**What are you good at?**

Using the ikigai model, start to make connections between the various lists looking for:

Passions: What you love and what you're good (enough) at.	Missions: What you love and what the world needs.
Vocations: What the world needs and what you can get paid for.	**Professions:** What you can get paid for and what you're good at.

Use this as a guide towards ideally finding a new ikigai (or composite ikigai), or at a minimum, finding a new vocation or profession to help meet your basic needs as the first step on your journey back up Maslow's Hierarchy.

Don't expect to find a job or activities to immediately replace the stimulus and reward of your military or first responder role after transition. It's likely that there will be a period of time when you feel unsettled no matter what you end up doing. A large part of this is due to the slowing of the pace of life when transitioning, which we'll take a deep dive into in the next chapter.

7. Your pace of life will slow.

I had anticipated my pace of life slowing down significantly as I approached transition and I had viewed this as a positive thing. While it was one of the few factors relating to discharge that I had considered consciously and understood in theory, I wasn't really prepared for the practical impact of the pace of my life slowing so rapidly.

To understand why a sudden slowing in the pace of life can feel so wrong, it's once again useful to go back to the start of a military or first responder career and track what is happening in the body's stress response system as an individual progresses in those roles.

On entry into the training pipeline for a military or first responder role it could be reasonably assumed that the trainee or recruit has lived a fundamentally normal life up until that point, and their stress response system has developed accordingly. What I mean by this is that their *subjective* experience of stress (how they consciously feel when they're stressed) is closely linked to their *objective* experience of stress (how their mind and body reacts to stress). If they encounter a sudden stressful situation, they will consciously register that it is indeed stressful and their body will react with increased heartrate, increased breathing rate, maybe sweating, anxiety, and perhaps fear or anger. How they consciously interpret the situation and how their body feels are aligned. If the situation is one of more chronic stress, such as the leadup to exams or the breakup of a relationship, likewise, they will usually be aware that they are stressed with signs such as irritability, poor sleep, and the like.

Once they hit the ground running for their training towards a military or first responder role the stress tap is turned on and it stays on. The initial shock and awe of the training will register consciously (holy fuck, what have I got myself into?) but after time they will adjust to the stress of their training and recalibrate to it. Before long the new, higher level of stress becomes their baseline and feels normal to them. Subjectively, they will no longer feel as consciously stressed as they had early in their training, but objectively the body is still experiencing the stress and upregulating its chronic stress response to keep the trainee ready to go at a moment's notice.

This process happens insidiously and continues throughout a career in a military or first responder role, with the individual generally being unaware of it occurring. The body starts to release slightly higher levels of a chronic stress hormone called cortisol, which peps us up and keeps us primed for action. Studies show that military members and first responders as groups have higher baseline levels of cortisol than people in other more *normal* jobs. This is an adaptive response, but over time can be quite damaging to the health of the individual who is chronically upregulated[13].

Just like a car engine that is constantly revving at five thousand revs and never returns to a low idle even when the car is stationary, the stress response systems of military members and first responders are constantly firing away.

It can be appreciated that a car engine that is always revving will wear out sooner and break down, and the exact same thing happens with people who are constantly firing their stress response system. This is one of the key factors that accounts for the higher rates of physical and mental health issues in career military and first responders when compared to other occupations.

Taking a step back from that point of breakdown, this chronic stress response is also what allows individuals in these roles to not only function but thrive in high stress conditions. And what's more, it can feel good!

Some will have heard of the *frog in boiling water*. The concept is that if you put a frog in cold water and then very gradually increase the heat, the frog doesn't register that the water is warming up and will stay in the pot until the water boils and the frog dies.

This can be used as an analogy for the slow and steady increase in stress in our lives not consciously registering and therefore not triggering us to feel the need to reduce

---

[13] For a deep dive into this concept, check out: van der Kolk, B. 2014, *The Body Keeps the Score*, Penguin Group, USA

or manage it until things hit crisis point. This is exactly what happens throughout a career in the military or a first responder role. The water is slowly warming up over the years, but we aren't noticing it. Another factor that compounds the situation is the fact that everyone else around us at work are in the same pot of slowly boiling water, so a reference point as to what a *normal* stress load looks like gets lost.

Let's fast forward now to transition out of a high stress role. The individual who has spent years to decades in an upregulated stress state (which they have recalibrated to and normalised) now finds themselves with far less stimulus to justify their stress, and they usually become immediately unsettled and bored shitless.

Another analogy that I think describes this period well is like having been driving on a highway for hours and hours at 110 kilometres per hour (about 68 miles per hour) and then having to slow down suddenly to 60 kph (37 mph to pass through a town), or worse, to 40kph (25mph) to pass through a school zone. Having adjusted to travelling at highway speeds it feels like the car is crawling along in a town or school speed limit.

This is exactly what happens during transition. The body's stress response has been upregulated to highway speeds and now you find yourself slowing down suddenly. Life feels intolerably slow, and your body is screaming at you to speed back up to feel *normal* again.

Back to the frog, this is the little critter hopping out of simmering water and immediately feeling uncomfortably cold. Its inclination is to want to hop straight back into the hot water that it has become used to.

Although it feels dreadful at the time, this reduction in stress is actually a good thing. If we allow ourselves to sit with the boredom and unease for long enough, our body's stress response system will most likely gradually wind back down and recalibrate to a healthier new normal state. Just like if we slowdown from the highway to town driving, after a while, driving at 60kph starts to feel normal again.

To be honest, the concept of allowing myself to be bored and to gradually adjust to a slower pace of life never even occurred to me when I transitioned out of the military. It was proposed to me about a year after my discharge when I was speaking with a trusted psychologist friend about how bored and unsettled I felt and everything I was doing to try to fill the stimulus void that was left after leaving the army. By that stage I was neck deep in university studies and had started several small businesses to try to warm the water back up to a point where I thought I would feel comfortable. The psychologist's advice was sage, but by the time I heard it I was already well committed in other areas and busy replacing my old stress with new stress.

Now I'm not suggesting that finding a new focus is a bad thing post-transition (in fact it's essential) however, I do urge people to consider what is happening from a stress response perspective and not just jump into the first available thing to provide stimulus to replace that from their old role.

At the risk of kicking the arse out of analogies in this

chapter, it can be like coming out of a long-term relationship and then jumping headfirst into a rebound relationship to fill the void. I think we'll all agree that the rebound lover is seldom *the one* and a bit of time spent single before committing again can provide some time for reflection and perspective before swiping right and getting back in the game!

Call to Action: Regulate your cortisol.

Cortisol is not a bad thing, it's only when it's released in abnormally high levels for long periods of time that it becomes toxic (like during a military or first responder career!). There's a bunch of things we can be doing to regulate our cortisol levels and help them wind back down to normal. Here's a few to consider:

- **Pay attention to your sleep.** Elevated cortisol and poor sleep go hand in hand. By paying close attention to your sleep, you can help reduce elevated cortisol and regulate it. Strategies to optimise sleep include[14]:
  o Limit alcohol
  o Limit caffeine – especially in the afternoon and evening
  o Limit nicotine – especially in the afternoon and evening
  o Try to stick to a regular bedtime – the body responds to consistency here
  o Use a sleep tracker to monitor how much of each

---

[14] For an online course focused on improving sleep in military and first responders, head to: https://aussiefrontline.com.au/courses/

sleep stage you're getting
- o Have a low-stimulus wind down routine at night
- o Avoid blue light exposure from screens for a couple of hours before bed
- o Keep your room as quiet, cool, and as dark as possible for sleep

- **Breathe.** Certain breathing patterns can help shut down your body's release of stress hormones such as cortisol and help activate your *rest and digest* (parasympathetic) nervous system. There are many you can search up, but here's a couple to get you started:
  - o **Box Breathing** – breathe in for four seconds, hold for four, breathe out for four, hold for four. Repeat
  - o **4-7-8 technique** – breathe in for four seconds, hold for seven, breathe out for eight. Repeat (no need to hold your breath after breathing out).

- **Pay attention to your diet.** Minimising processed foods and those high in sugar has been linked with cortisol reduction.

- **Exercise regularly.** There are endless types of exercise, all with their own pros and cons. I recommend finding whatever works for you and do it regularly but not to extremes. Also, try to avoid vigorous exercise close to bedtime, as it can wind you up and make it harder to get to sleep. If it suits your routine to exercise close to bedtime, try light exercise such as yoga or stretching.

- **Journal.** Several studies have shown that regular journaling can reduce cortisol levels. It's also a great way to get your thoughts out on paper and help to make sense of the transition period with a view to moving forward in a positive fashion.

- **Practice gratitude.** The simple act of deliberately focusing on the positive things in our life has been linked to reduced cortisol levels. Due to their training and exposures, military members and first responders can become accustomed to looking for and focusing on the negatives in life. This is a normal adaptive response to the roles, and it can take dedicated practice to look hard for, and focus on, positives.

- **Get a hobby.** Look for an outlet that you enjoy and get involved. A great place to start is the list of missions and passions you created in Chapter 6.

- **Meditate.** Often meditation is dismissed as not relevant in military and first responder cultures, but nothing could be further from the truth. Meditation is a superpower and is a proven technique to downregulate abnormally elevated cortisol levels, as well as reduce acute stress response reactions (fight or flight). The bottom line is that meditation not only regulates chronic stress but makes you a better operator in acute stress situations, allowing you to think more clearly and perform at a higher level.

A good place to start is one of the many guided meditation apps. When starting off it's important to remember that your mind will wander all the time, it's programmed to do this. This doesn't mean your failing at meditation, the process that leads to adaptation over time is catching your brain wandering and bringing it back to focus. This is like doing a rep for your brain. The ability to quiet your mind is the end state of deliberate practice of meditation over time. It doesn't take hours and hours of training to have an effect, as little as 10-12 minutes a day, done most days, will start to downregulate your stress response within a couple of weeks.

- **Pat a pet.** There's some great evidence to show that hanging out with a pet reduces stress levels. Studies suggest that dogs are the way to go here, but I reckon time with any pet will do.

- **Hang out with mates.** Social interaction is an age-old technique for releasing feel good chemicals into our systems and reducing stress. If you can be doing something outdoors in nature, then that has been shown to amplify the positive effect.

Need a buzz?

If you are climbing the walls in transition and feel the need to get a stress hormone hit, it's important to do it in an adaptive way. If you're planning on replacing stimulus long term, try to plan your activities to align with something that you feel might be a productive commitment to work towards rebuilding the upper layers of your Maslow's Hierarchy and ideally move you towards ikigai. Try to resist the urge to jump at the first thing that comes along just to feel stimulated again.

For adaptive ways to get a quick stress hormone fix, here's a couple of things to try:

- Intensive exercise. Something like a High Intensity Interval Training (HIIT) session fits the bill here.

- Cold water immersion. Start with a blast of cold water in the shower and work your way up to ice baths if you dare!

One final way to regulate cortisol levels (and potentially get a controlled stress hormone hit) is to engage in what's known as *flow state* activities, which just so happens to be the topic of the next chapter.

8. You will lose your flow

The flow state is something that most will be familiar with, but once again, may not have had cause to think deeply about. It is often referred to as *being in the zone* and describes a mental state where, under the right conditions, you become completely immersed in what you are doing.

One of the hallmarks of flow is the distortion of our perception of time, most commonly the sensation that time has flown by when we emerge back out of flow state. It might have felt like you've only spent 15 minutes doing an activity, but when you check your watch, you realise that an hour has passed. This distortion of time is caused by a change in the pathways that are firing in your brain when you experience flow and a downregulation of activity in the region of the brain that keeps track of time. More rarely, time can seem to slow during intensely engaging experiences but typically it seems to speed up. Although you're not often aware of having a positive experience when you're in the flow state (due to the downregulation of neural pathways that track your sense of pleasure), the aftermath of flow is often invigorating. You can be left feeling on a high and buzzing for hours.

The main man responsible for the original research into the flow state, and the guy who coined the term, was the fantastically named Hungarian American psychologist Mihaly Csikszentmihalyi (last name pronounced roughly *chick-sent-me-hi*).

As a funny aside, I was once presenting on resilience to a hospitality group and there was a particular gentleman in the audience who appeared to be a little worse for wear. I would later find out that he was nursing a whopping hangover from some birthday celebrations the night before. The rest of the audience was pleasingly engaged, but this poor bloke was obviously hanging by a thread and drifting in and out of consciousness throughout the session. During a break shortly after discussing the flow state and mentioning Csikszentmihalyi's name, the bloke approached me and asked, "what was that you said about *chicks in knee-highs*?". I digress, back to the point.

Csikszentmihalyi describes 8 characteristics of flow[15]:

1. Complete concentration on the task;
2. Clarity of goals and reward in mind, with immediate feedback;
3. Transformation of time (speeding up/slowing down);
4. The experience is intrinsically rewarding;

[15] Csikszentmihalyi, M. 2008. Flow: The psychology of optimal experience. Perennial, USA.

5. Effortlessness and ease;
6. There is a balance between challenge and skills;
7. Actions and awareness are merged, losing self-conscious rumination;
8. There is a feeling of control over the task.

With hindsight, I realise that my military career was full of opportunities to tap into flow states. Initially this occurred in my training pipeline as I was required to learn new skills at a rapid rate, forcing me to fully engage and immerse myself in the learning process. Then, as my career progressed I had more and more opportunities to find flow in both my military and medical duties.

The key to clicking your brain into a flow state is to be performing an activity right around the limits of your current ability to do it. If the activity is too easy for your ability, then boredom occurs, and flow can't be achieved. On the other end of the spectrum, if the activity is too hard, you can't get in the zone due to anxiety and frustration at the inability to perform it. It needs to be right in that sweet spot for your skill level at that particular time.

This highlights another fantastic thing to know about flow, you don't need to be particularly good at the activity to tap into a flow state. You simply need to be doing it at the level of your current skill level.

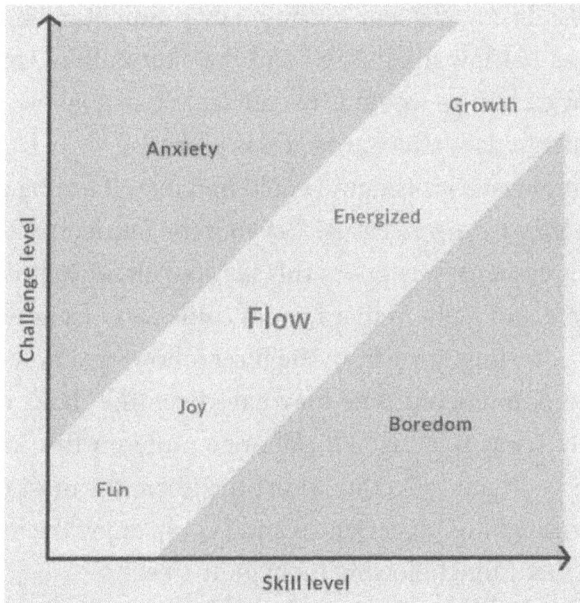

Figure 9. Flow states occur when the challenge of an activity and current skill levels are well matched. (Image source: www.PositivePsychology.com)

As my skills progressed throughout my military career, I was able to find flow in more and more complex situations. The ultimate environment for me was combat, and specifically treating combat casualties on the battlefield. Once I had reached the appropriate level of competence to conduct myself appropriately on the battlefield, and to have the skills readily available to me to approach a combat casualty with confidence, the stage was set for some of my most epic flow state experiences.

I was in my element in those environments (self-actu-alised as Maslow might say!) and the aftermath of treating combat casualties would leave me feeling as high as a kite for hours to days afterwards. It was addictive.

Somewhat confusingly, I could find myself feeling exhil-arated after treating a casualty even if the ultimate outcome for that casualty was poor. This led to a significant degree of shame and guilt, in that I could come away from the ex-perience feeling great from the buzz following a flow state, but the ultimate outcome may have been the death of the casualty I was treating (I'll elaborate more on this in later chapters). Thankfully, this wasn't the norm for most of my work-related flow experiences and I could enjoy the invigo-ration that came following them guilt-free.

It wasn't until I discharged from the army that I came to realise that I didn't have any flow state activities outside of work. I simply hadn't felt the need to pursue any due to the itch being scratched regularly at work.

With hindsight, the absence of flow was yet another negative aspect of my transition back to civilian life that compounded the perceived boredom and dissatisfaction I felt during the transition period. I eventually realised that finding some new flow-state activities would be a great thing to do, but I had become programmed to associate them with high-octane military or medical experiences. It took me quite some time to realise that I needed to broaden the lens a little to find flow.

There's no question that you can find flow in adrenaline-fuelled activities such as skydiving, motorsports, and downhill mountain bike riding, and often these are natural go-to flow state activities for transitioning military members and first responders. They are culturally aligned with the mindset of those organisations and if those pursuits are of interest to you, then go for broke with them (but try not to get broken while doing them!).

If, like me, you don't necessarily find yourself craving the adrenaline of these type of activities, you can still definitely find flow in more sedate pursuits. As stated above, you just need to be doing the activity around the level of your current competence and you can find flow.

Another couple of hacks to facilitate flow states are to minimise potential distractions (set your phone to silent, stick some headphones in and play some tunes, or let others know you don't want to be disturbed if appropriate) and also to set a timeframe to complete an activity within. For the right activities, these two additional considerations can significantly increase the chance of achieving a flow state.

From there, the sky is pretty much the limit for finding flow. Every time I present to an audience on flow, I put it out to the room to tell me their flow state activities. There's always a few left-of-centre ones, but the following are regular responses:

- Exercise such as running, riding a bike, swimming laps
- Riding a motorbike or driving a car
- Working on a motorbike or car (or any other form of machinery)

- Surfing or sailing
- Rock-climbing, abseiling, mountaineering
- Fishing, hunting, or shooting
- Reading a book
- Mowing the lawn or gardening
- Playing with a dog or riding a horse
- Listening to music, playing a musical instrument, or writing music (if you're that talented!)
- Cooking, and even cleaning the house – vacuuming, mopping, or dusting
- Drawing, painting, pottery, or any other similar creative outlet
- Woodwork, metalwork, or similar creative endeavours that use your hands
- Doing jigsaw puzzles, Suduko and other similar puzzles, or playing boardgames
- Creative writing

The list goes on and is only limited by your personal preferences and imagination. Remember, you don't need to be good at the activity to tap into flow, you just need to be doing it at the level of your competence.

Also, flow state activities are not about the outcome, they are about the process. I've spent many hours immersed in flow to pop out at the other end with a complete piece of shit metal or woodwork project, or an inedible meal when cooking. While it's always nice to have something to show for your efforts, the real reward is the mental health benefits of the flow state itself.

On a physiological level, there's some compelling evidence to show that regularly tapping into flow helps to regulate cortisol levels, as well as reduce what's known as the Default Mode Network (DMN), commonly referred to as the *monkey mind*, being the pesky loops of almost always negative thoughts that play in our mind when it's not meaningfully occupied. The monkey mind has a habit of being in overdrive during the transition period and fuels the chronic stress response. Anything you can be doing to quieten the monkey down a little is a hugely positive thing.

Call to Action: Find your flow

Complete the following table:

	Activity
What flow-state activities did you have in your old role that you will lose access to after transition?	
What flow-state activities from your old role might you be able to continue post-transition?	

What flow-state activities do you do outside of work that you can continue post-transition?	
Are there flow-state activities that you used to do but have stopped doing during your old role? Maybe it's time to start them up again!	
What new flow-state activities would you be interested in exploring post-transition?	

Maybe some of these activities might fit neatly into the *passions* section of the ikigai construct (although you don't need to be good at them to find flow). For extra marks, look for flow state activities that you might be able to do with others to create the opportunity to make new friend-ships (and rebuild the psychological layer of your Maslow's Hierarchy) or perhaps even find a new tribe.

In the next chapter, we're going to explore our tendency to look back on things with fondness. So, chuck on your rose-coloured glasses and keep reading!

9. You'll look back with rose coloured glasses

For a couple of years after my transition out of the army I wished I could go back. For all the reasons discussed so far in this book, I was unsettled, understimulated, and struggling to find a new purpose and identity.

Around the two-year mark I had started to make progress in the right direction thanks to taking a job in a small regional hospital as their Deputy Medical Superintendent. The Superintendent was an old army mate of mine which definitely helped, but it was more than that. I was once again part of a small, hard-working team, and could feel a sense of significance and purpose returning. I was most of the way through studying my Master of Business Administration (MBA) and was putting the management and leadership skills that I was learning into practice in my new role.

From a medical skill perspective, I was once again on a steep learning curve, re-learning old medical skills that I hadn't really needed in the military, such as looking after kids, elderly, and those with chronic illnesses, as well as extending my emergency medicine skills in areas other than trauma. All of this was contributing significantly to me rebuilding the psychological layers of my Maslow's Hierarchy.

The hospital only had six doctors on the roster, meaning that we worked closely and experienced ups and downs together, creating the beginnings of a new sense of tribe. Involvement in the occasional life and death resuscitation situation in the emergency department of the hospital even allowed me to recapture some of the stimulus and access to flow states that I had missed so much from my military days of treating combat casualties. I was well and truly starting to rebuild myself, and yet when I reflected on my army days, a big part of me regretted discharging and still craved being back there.

Things changed around that time due to a chance encounter with a couple of old army special operations colleagues. I had randomly bumped into them in an airport lounge, and I learned that they were soon to conduct a training exercise in the town where I was living. They had been on a reconnaissance trip to set up contacts and plan logistics for the training exercise and were still looking for a few additional business contacts in the area, which I helped them out with.

It was during my interactions with these old army mates of mine that I had an epiphany.

It occurred to me that they were still doing the exact same things that they had been doing while I was at the unit. In effect, they were basically living the same year, year after year. Don't get me wrong, it was still appealing and exciting to me, but what I could suddenly see was the fact that I had progressed and evolved from my former military self. I was most of the way through my MBA, I had evolved as a doctor, and as a leader in my hospital role. Things that wouldn't have happened if I'd stayed in the army.

For the first time since I transitioned out of the army, I realised with clarity that I had made the correct decision. I was growing as a person, and it felt great. I could also see with clarity that I had started to stagnate in my old military role, yet when I had previously reflected, I had tended only to reminisce on the good parts of the job. I never seemed to reflect on all the negatives, of which there were many. Somehow, they didn't seem to feature in my memories, but the interactions with my former colleagues for some reason allowed me to have a far more balanced recollection of my army role.

Rosy Retrospection

It turns out that the tendency to look back on the *good old days* of our lives with *rose coloured glasses* is a normal human bias. The psychologists call this bias *rosy retrospection*[16], and it causes us to perceive the past as better than it was, which can then have the effect of diminishing our present experience in comparison.

This distorted perspective can compound all the other

---

[16] For more on Rosy Retrospection, check out: www.thedecisionlab.com

stresses faced during transition significantly, to the point where individuals can actually *grieve* the loss of their *perception* of their former self. It probably plays a decent role in the decision that some make to go back to their previous jobs, perhaps only to find themselves then realising that it wasn't quite what they remembered it to be. This is because it wasn't the job as they remembered it, they had been misled by rosy retrospection!

Another interesting aspect of rosy retrospection is what is known as the *reminiscence bump*, which is a period of our lives that research suggests is when we form our most vivid long-term memories. This period is centred around ages 20-30 and it is believed that higher concentrations of neurotransmitters such as dopamine in our brains at that age cause us to form more vivid memories from that period than from other stages of our lives.

When we consider that age period of intensified memory formation, it can be appreciated that it occurs when most military members and first responders are entering into their role, becoming indoctrinated into their tribe, and starting to have the rich and unique experiences that the roles offer.

Compounding the positive distortion of rosy retrospection is often photos and other memorabilia of service, that mostly reflect good experiences from the role. Photos with mates, at graduations and perhaps award ceremonies, and other significant positive moments. It's less likely that the photos taken, and memorabilia kept and reflected on, are those from traumatic or negative experiences.

In their *transition stress* article (which if you haven't yet read, you must!) Mobbs & Bonanno[17] discuss the concept of autobiographical memories (AM) and momentous events serving as transition points and acting as *bookends* to distinct periods of our life. These momentous events in the life of a military member or first responder include entry into and transition out of the role. In relation to military members specifically (but equally applicable to first responders), Mobbs & Bonanno state:

> "As transitions serve to organize AM and turning points anchor the life story, entry in to and exit out of military service potentially creates watershed moments which serve to accentuate the period in between".

It turns out that there is some science behind the tongue-in-cheek saying *the older I get, the better I was*. However, this perception of how good you may have been, as well as how good things were, when you were younger is distorted in a positive fashion. None the less, it can lead to a very real experience of grieving your former self.

---

[17] Mobbs MC, Bonanno GA. Beyond war and PTSD: The crucial role of transition stress in the lives of military veterans. Clin Psychol Rev. 2018 Feb;59:137-144. doi: 10.1016/j.cpr.2017.11.007. Epub 2017 Nov 21.

Grieving your former self

Turning our attention to grief, there's some well-defined stages associated with the emotion. I certainly experienced all of these to some degree during my transition out of the army and reassimilation into civilian life. Once again, there's different models of the grief process, but I'm going to use the 5-Stage model developed by Swiss psychiatrist Elisabeth Kubler-Ross[18].

Stages of grief.
1. Denial
2. Anger
3. Bargaining
4. Depression
5. Acceptance

Kubler-Ross' work was initially related to grief following the death of a loved one; however, her model has been widely applied to any significant life change and an adaptation is graphically represented as the Kubler-Ross Change Curve (Figure 10), which I think is applicable to transition.

---

[18] Kubler-Ross, E. 1969. *On Death and Dying.* 1st Edn., Macmillan, New York.

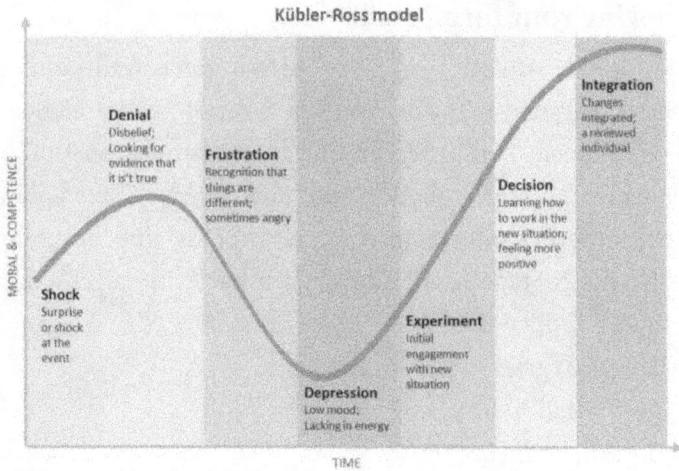

Figure 10. Kubler-Ross Change Curve. (Image source: www.clever-ism.com)

My transition followed this exact emotional roller-coaster ride. I initially experienced a brief upturn in my wellbeing when I transitioned due to an exclusive focus on the positives that came with it. I felt as though the weight of my military role had been suddenly lifted and that my civilian future was full of exciting future potential. Although I of course knew I had discharged from the army, a large part of me was in denial and it felt initially like I was just on a period of extended leave and that I would ultimately return to the role.

For me, this first *honeymoon* phase of relative positivity lasted about six months, and it was at that point I started the downturn of frustration and into the depression stage of Kubler-Ross' Change Curve.

The subsequent experiment phase involved a trial-and-error period of trying on some new civilian identities (attempting to resolve my identity crisis). I had a bit of a false start as a fly-in, fly-out, doctor on a mine site before finding a new identity that seemed to fit (working in the regional hospital). From there, the uptick of the Change Curve really gained momentum and I was able to achieve my new identity, start to rebuild the upper layers of my Maslow's Hierarchy, and power forward through the decision and integration stages of the Change Curve.

It's important to appreciate that all of this takes time. While everyone is different, and it's not possible to put defined timeframes on any given stage of the grief process or the Change Curve model, the stages are generally measured in months as opposed to weeks and the whole process can be reasonably expected to take years.

The key take-home points from this chapter are that after transitioning you will probably reflect on your former role with the falsely positive distortion of rosy retrospection and that you are likely to ride the emotional rollercoaster of the Kubler-Ross Change Curve as you grieve the loss of your former self. This rollercoaster ride will take months to years, will probably have a brief upward phase, before plummeting down into a period of depression, but, with effort, will then head back up again to a better place.

Call to action: Take off the rose coloured glasses!

In this activity, list the positive recollections from your previous role, but also list the negatives. The goal here is to defeat the tendency towards rosy retrospection and provide a more balanced memory of how the job actually was.

What was good about the role?	What about the role sucked?

Call to action: Ride the Kubler-Ross Rollercoaster.

Take another look at the Kubler-Ross Change Curve.

If you've already transitioned out of your former role, can you identify where you are at on the curve?

If you're about to transition, create the expectation that things will get worse before they get better as you grieve your former self.

Whatever stage you're at, know that ultimately there is a positive endpoint, but it will take some work to get there and there will be some tough times on the way. It's also likely that you'll experience loneliness during transition, which is the topic of the next chapter.

10. You will be lonely

Loneliness is a killer. Literally.

In our book *The Resilience Shield*[19], we cite studies led by US Surgeon General Vivek Murthy declaring loneliness as a public health epidemic in the United States and linking the negative health effects of being lonely to the equivalent of smoking 15 cigarettes a day!

Underpinning the negative physical health effects of loneliness is the increased release of chronic stress hormones that results from not being socially connected and supported. As mentioned in Chapter 4, from an evolutionary perspective, dislocation from our tribe meant an increased risk of death from exposure, predators, or starvation, and hence drove a significant stress response. While those threats don't exist to the same degree as they once did, the physiological stress response to loneliness remains very real and dangerous.

Loneliness is an unpleasant emotional reaction to

[19] Pronk D, Pronk B, and Curtis T, 2021, *The Resilience Shield*, Macmillan Australia, Sydney.

perceived isolation. The word *perceived* here is important, because it's possible to feel lonely even when surrounded by people. During my period of transition from the army I came across this quote about loneliness from 20th century Swiss psychiatrist Carl Jung (more from him later), that resonated deeply:

"Loneliness does not come from having no people about one, but from being unable to communicate the things that seem important to oneself, or from holding certain views which others find inadmissible".

During my transition I was surrounded by people, yet I felt intensely lonely. I was no longer part of the military tribe that I had become identity fused with, and my opinions and values at the time were so profoundly misaligned with the civilians that I found myself associating with that I didn't feel I could connect with them on any level. It was as though they were a different species.

I recall one specific instance, around nine months into my transition, when I found myself at a social gathering with a group of my wife's friends and their husbands or partners. After a few brief (and admittedly feeble) attempts at engaging socially, I quickly gave up and retreated to a corner to drink my beer alone. Scanning the crowd, I remember judging them one by one in my mind; dickhead, dickhead, dickhead, and on I went as my eyes moved from one person to the next.

It was during this harsh and ignorant mental judgement session that I had an epiphany. It was highly improbable that everyone at the gathering except me was a dickhead. If there was a Bell Curve placed over society with dickheads at the extreme left and good blokes (and girls) at the extreme right, then statistically it was nearly impossible that the group I was scanning were all dickheads. It became abundantly clear that the problem was me and if there was a dickhead in the room, then it was me!

More likely, there were no dickheads present that night, the issue was not one of dickheadedness, but rather of disconnection. I was experiencing the sense of loneliness described by Jung in which I felt unable to communicate things that seemed important to me with the other partygoers and feared that my views may be inadmissible to them.

I still identified as part of the military in-group (which by definition I wasn't any longer) and found myself at a gathering of civilians (that I still psychologically considered an out-group). I was in the depths of the *depression* stage of Kubler-Ross' Change Curve and yet to reach the uptick of the *experiment* stage, where I would eventually start to engage with my new situation and make positive efforts to integrate with the civilian in-group. All of this fuelled my loneliness.

Once again, as with most things psychological and scientific, there are multiple tools that can be used to quantify loneliness. The one that I find most useful is the UCLA loneliness scale. It's a 20-question survey with response options ranging from *never* to *always*. Here's a snapshot of the questions in the survey:

1. How often do you feel that you are "in tune" with the people around you?
2. How often do you feel part of a group of friends?
3. How often do you feel that you have a lot in common with the people around you?
4. How often do you feel that your interests and ideas are not shared by those around you?
5. How often do you feel left out?
6. How often do you feel that no one really knows you well?

If you've recently transitioned from the military or a first responder role, I can pretty much guarantee that you will answer *never* to questions 1,2, and 3, and *always* to questions 4,5, and 6. If I had done the UCLA Loneliness Score on the night I found myself at the social gathering described above, I would have scored off the scale. From a physical health perspective, I might as well have been in the corner chain-smoking a pack of cigarettes with my beer!

Integration into new groups and new identity achievement takes time (usually years) and deliberate effort. Normally, the unique factors that facilitated your former military or first responder identity are not present. You're not forced into groups with people and there's no shared goals and suffering to expedite and strengthen group formation. You need to seek out new groups and actively pursue integration. You generally won't feel like doing this, however you must.

Other indices of loneliness use questions relating to how often you talk to, or get together with, family, friends, or neighbours, and how often you attend meetings of clubs or organisations you belong to. These questions highlight the clues as to how to cure loneliness, you need to engage and seek out new friendships and tribes. Look for passions and missions (from the ikigai concept) and potentially for flow state opportunities through hobby groups and sporting team affiliation. If you're religious (or would consider it), get to a place of worship.

In the years that followed by transition out of the army (and after my realisation that civilians were not a lesser species with an overrepresentation of dickheads among them) I became far more proactive in my efforts to build new friendships.

I started to see the process as a game of *Social UNO*, let me explain.

Most will be familiar with the card game UNO, if you're not that's ok, the basic premise is easily understood. Most of the deck of UNO cards have a number on them (0-9) and are either red, yellow, green, or blue in colour. There are some funky cards with different functions, but for the purposes of this analogy let's ignore those.

The game begins with an initial card being laid down and then, where possible, players put a card of matching number or colour on top of it. When it comes to applying this to a social interaction, it's all about looking for common interests or values with those you're interacting with. You don't need to match them perfectly in these departments (both number and colour don't need to match!), you just need to look for a common thread and pursue it. Sometimes this is easier said than done, and sometimes this isn't possible, but I find it to be a good starting point when I'm meeting people for the first time who I don't obviously have anything in common with.

For example, one particular husband of a friend of my wife was a former professional football player and a football coach at the time of my transition. I don't particularly care about football and, our previous roles of professional football and special operations doctoring seemed fairly disparate. Over time however, we bonded over a shared interest in high performance teams, and I even went on to run a leadership development program for up-and-coming leaders in his football team, based on military leadership principles that worked well in the army.

Another example was with a bloke who ran a blind man-ufacturing company. Now I'm not sure that you could find a more different role than that from army special operations, however when we scratched the surface, we found a shared interest in all things related to running a small business, as well as a shared love for cars.

My point is this; if you actually make the effort to engage with people and look for shared interests and values (play Social UNO), more often than not you will find them. Those people may not end up being lifelong buddies or members of your future tribe, but unless you make the effort, you will never know. I've certainly had plenty of social situations since transitioning from the army where I have simply not been able to find any common ground with people. That's normal, and in that setting it's perfectly fine to throw down a wildcard and leave the conversation!

A great technique to use when playing Social UNO is active listening. Once again, we cover this skill in *The Resilience Shield* as a strategy to help build your Social Layer. Active listening involves listening attentively to the person speaking (rather than just watching for their lips to stop moving and waiting eagerly for your turn to talk) and then responding by reflecting on what has been said (paraphrase their words back to them) and retaining the information for use later in the conversation as appropriate.

As a generalisation, people love to talk about themselves and by using active listening they are likely to keep talking and giving you a greater opportunity of finding out a common interest that you can latch on to.

All of this is probably the last thing you feel like doing when you're grieving your former self, you've lost the upper layers of your Maslow's Hierarchy, ikigai seems like a distant memory (if you ever achieved it), and you're bottoming out in the depression stage of Kubler-Ross' Change Curve. But remember the sage words of Marcus Aurelius, you must:

"…get active in your own rescue".

Call to action: Know your enemy – Loneliness

Quantify your loneliness using the UCLA Loneliness Scale (find it using an internet search). Depending on where you're at in your transition process, you might score highly on this scale. Don't despair, it's only a snapshot of where you are currently at and a starting point for the pathway forward in building new social connections.

Call to action: Practice Active Listening.

To get started on this one, try a trick used by hostage negotiators around the world, known as *mirroring*. Simply repeat the last three words of any sentence someone says to you, or the three key words from what they've said. From there, pause and wait for them to keep talking. It's nothing short of a Jedi mind trick.

Once you latch on to a common interest in the conversation, play Social UNO and take the conversation in that direction.

11. Your old values may no longer serve you

My first car was a real piece of shit, but I loved it. It was a bright yellow 1977 Triumph 2500 TC and I recall specifically that it cost $1250 (albeit in 1996). I owned that car for about five years and over that time I sunk what little cash I had into restoring it and, where possible, improving it. I rebuilt the carburettors, replaced fuel pumps and starter motors, and made sure it always had fresh spark plugs, oil, and oil and petrol filters. Mechanically, it was great, but over the years I owned it, it developed a serious rust problem. What started as a few bubbles here and there progressed rapidly to be structural issues as the metal cancer took hold. Eventually it became clear that while the engine was going strong, the body of the car was unsalvageable.

The answer was obvious to me; remove the engine and other good bits from the old, rusted car (including the amps and four subwoofers that I had installed in the boot by that stage), get myself another Triumph 2500 with a decent body, and put it all together to make a drivable car. The old car wasn't saleable in its rusted state as it couldn't be registered, but it didn't make sense to throw the baby out with the bathwater and scrap the whole thing as some of the parts were perfectly good for ongoing road use (and doof-doof noise pollution).

I have come to see this example as analogous to my values when I left the army. At the time of my transition, I had a rigid set of values that had served me very well in the military, but I had failed to consider that the exact same values may not be perfectly suited to civilian life. Indeed, some of them would prove to be completely misaligned to civilian life, but no one ever told me that, and I didn't think to consider it until years after I discharged.

Metaphorically, some of my values were like the rusted shell of my old Triumph and needed to be thrown away. Others were like the strong engine (and thumping sub-woofers) of the old beast and could be kept and inserted into my new civilian identity to power forward with.

In Chapter 3 we discussed values and hopefully you took the time to either look up a list of common values and scribble down a few that resonate, or to do the Values Project survey[20]. The goal there was to better know yourself, with a view to looking for potential work and other endeavours that align with your personal values. In this chapter, the intent is to elaborate a little on values and get you to challenge the appropriateness of your current values during transition out of a military or first responder role.

---

[20] www.thevaluesproject.com

Values can and do change over time. It's likely that you will have some hardwired values, known as *core values*, that are far less likely to change over time. However, we also have what's known as *derived*, or *secondary values*, that still contribute to making us the unique people we are but are far more amenable to change over time.

When you stop to think about it, you are still fundamentally the same person that you were as a teenager, however the things you value will likely have changed significantly through your adult lives. For example, I no longer value rendering myself (and anyone else in the grid square) deaf from blasting doof-doof music from multiple subwoofers in my car. During my military career, I found that gunfire and being in close proximity to blasts was a way of achieving the same outcome that was more aligned with my values at the time!

All jokes aside, our values can, and do, change over time and what's more, we can actively change them if we identify ones that no longer serve us well in the life stage we find ourselves in. This is likely going to be the case when transitioning out of military and first responder roles.

There will be certain values that an individual has that probably led them to enter a military or first responder role in the first place. From there, the individual is indoctrinated into the organisational values, commonly including those on the following list:

- Courage
- Respect

- Integrity
- Excellence
- Service
- Leadership
- Collaboration
- Ongoing learning

These are all excellent values to have and should be kept throughout the transition period and onward in life. Other values may not be as well suited to life post service. A few values that I eventually realised were counterproductive after my discharge from the army, and the reasons why, are listed below:

Elite physical fitness.

Throughout my army career I had strived to maintain elite levels of physical fitness. This was initially essential in preparing for, and passing, SAS selection. From there, it was necessary to maintain a very high level of fitness to do my role. It wasn't uncommon to find myself lugging around a combat load upwards of 50kg (110 pounds), often at altitude in places like Afghanistan, and over mountainous terrain.

When we were back home in barracks, our normal work day allowed us a couple of hours for physical training and when we were deployed, one of the highest priorities, wherever we found ourselves, was to set up a gym so we could keep training. Physical fitness was ingrained in the culture and values of the unit.

It didn't occur to me until years after discharge that I didn't need to maintain the same rate of effort with my physical training, and indeed it had started to become counterproductive. Not only was the rate of effort requiring me to find time in my week around new work commitments (eating into my family time), but my aging body was also starting to show signs of wear and tear.

The realisation that I needed to wind back my training came about five years after my discharge, when I had set myself the goal of a 200kg (440 pound) deadlift and a 100kg (220 pound) clean and jerk. Weighing around 70kg (155 pounds) myself at the time and creeping into my mid-40s, my body let me know it wasn't happy with these pursuits through a bulged spinal disc rubbing on nerves and giving me hellish sciatica.

Predictably, I initially chewed anti-inflammatories (the culturally appropriate management of any injury in the army) and trained through it for a few months before the pain became unmanageable and I was forced to reassess my goals. A spinal surgeon reinforced this recommendation and convinced me to adopt a more age and stage appropriate fitness regime. The reality was that I had absolutely no *need* to be lifting those sorts of weights, but it had been programmed into my values in the military and I hadn't considered winding it back on discharge.

Relentless pursuit of excellence.

Another value that was inherent to army special operations was the *relentless pursuit of excellence*. This worked brilliantly in that environment and kept every member of the unit striving to be their individual best and to push the organisational capability to excellence.

This value works well in organisations where everyone has been specifically selected for their role and are passionately united towards a common mission. This value did continue to serve me well in my medical leadership role in the small hospital I worked at for a few years post-discharge, as the team there was small, focussed, and invested in personal and organisational excellence. It was only when I was three years out of the army that it started to become clear that I needed to soften that particular value.

By that stage, I had moved into another medical management role as the Medical Director for a State-wide medical capability. It was a much larger team than the one we had in the small hospital, and there were far more political and logistical constraints. The end result was a slower moving machine whose operational outputs were generally only at the functional level at best. Many of the staff that I worked alongside, as well as those I managed, didn't value the relentless pursuit of excellence that I had become accustomed to in the military, and saw their roles more as a vocation or profession (remember the ikigai diagram).

This is of course perfectly fine, and the reality is that most people in the broader population will approach their work with this mindset, however, for me at the time it created significant frustration and value incongruence. I could see some clear areas where the organisation could improve, but no matter how much energy I invested, I was just one tiny cog in a massive machine. I could spin and spin as fast as I was capable of but if the other cogs weren't spinning at the same rate, then my efforts were futile.

I began to see that my individual relentless pursuit of excellence was only serving to create frustration and burn me out, with no improvement in organisational capability. As defeatist as it felt at the time, I resigned myself to backing off a little and only investing the appropriate amount of energy into the role that was commensurate with all of those around me. It was this very realisation, that my values were incongruent with those of the broader organisation, that would eventually lead me to resign from the role.

Punctuality.

As I'm sure most former military and first responders will attest to, punctuality is crucial in those roles. Being late simply isn't a thing, and for good reason. If you're late to a house fire as a firefighter, a heart attack as a paramedic, a street brawl as a police officer, or a helicopter extraction on operations as a military member, the outcome could quite literally be fatal. If you're late to a Commanding Officer's set of orders, the outcome may not be literally fatal, but you may find yourself wising you were dead!

There is a saying in the army that goes; *if you're not ten early, you're ten late.*

The value of punctuality is drilled into military members and first responders during their initial training and maintained throughout their careers. The reality, however, is that outside of those lines of work, it often really doesn't matter that much if you're a little late for something. It's impolite and sometimes disrespectful, but it's not life and death. Yet many ex-military and first responders (myself included) rigidly carry this value with them after transition and apply it to all aspects of their lives.

I have insight into it now, but I continue to find my blood pressure rising when my wife is still doing her makeup as the time we were meant to meet friends has ticked past. Surprisingly, me checking my watch every 30 seconds, and encouraging her to hurry up, generally doesn't help the situation! I still firmly believe that punctuality is a great value to have, and it's one I continue to attempt to instil into my kids (and with lesser success, my wife) however, I have finally realised that continuing to hold the value of military-grade punctuality is not useful as a civilian.

Prioritising the mission over all else.

This is a somewhat unique value that is only really held by military and first response organisations. When you think about it, what other roles would ask to you potentially risk your life in the line of duty?

A brief scrub of the internet reveals this value reflected in organisational statements such as the following:

Service – The selflessness of character to place the security and interests of our nation and its people ahead of one's own. Australian Army

Loyalty – Devote yourself to the U.S. Constitution, the Army, your unit, and other fellow Soldiers. US Army

Service – We are devoted to serving our community with honour, placing the needs of the community above those of our own. Windsor Police

Patient First – Our patients are at the centre of everything we do. South Australian Ambulance Service

Putting communities first – Firefighters are expected to put the interests of the public, their community, and service users first at all times - UK Fire and Rescue Service

And probably most concisely and impactfully put:

Semper Fidelis (always faithful) - US Marine Corps moto

These are powerful values that every member of the respective organisation strives to uphold. They also serve to bond the tribe together and facilitate the in-group strength that leads to identity fusion. The visceral sense of oneness that comes with identity fusion is what ultimately reinforces the sense of loyalty, service, and duty, that allows the individual members of the organisation to reach the point where they would willingly risk their lives for the mission, their teammates, or the general community. It is essential to the individual and collective objectives of military and first response organisations, but it often comes at the cost of relationships with family and friends outside of work.

There's another saying that goes; *if the army wanted you to have a family, they would have issued you with one!*

I'm sure that similar sayings exist in other military and first responder organisations, and the truth that underpins it is universal. When we consider those in our society who have more *normal* jobs, it is far less likely that they will experience the same degree of in-group bonding with their work teams and therefore would be significantly less likely to become identity fused in their role. Their best chance of experiencing identity fusion will be with their family and perhaps close friends. That is what normal looks like.

When a military member or first responder becomes identity fused with their work role, this becomes direct competition to their identity fusion with their family unit. Birthdays and Christmases are routinely missed due to work commitments, as are births of children, trips to the emergency department for broken bones and cut knees, and the list goes on. This is how it must be, and most members can justify missing these key life events due to their level of investment in their role.

While this level of investment might be required during service, I believe the value of prioritising work over family is one that is counterproductive post-transition, and a reca-libration is required. I realised this too late.

In my book *The Combat Doctor*, I tell the story of how, without resentment, I blame the army for my failure to see my dying dad one last time.

I was three years out of uniform by that time, so I certainly couldn't blame the Green-Machine directly for having me deployed or otherwise committed at the time. The issue was that my mindset was still of prioritisation of the mission above all else.

I was mid-way through a block of shifts in the emergency department of the regional hospital I was helping to run when my dad's health began to deteriorate sharply. He had been battling cancer for years by that point and it was clear that he was in his final days. Rather than drop everything and get to his bedside like a normal son would, I planned to finish my block of shifts and then visit dad on my days off. Dad passed away prior to that.

It would take another couple of years to finally recali-brate my *mission-first* values to the more appropriate *family-first* values. That day finally came when one of my sons broke a finger and I left work instantly to be by his side at the hospital for his management and then grab some Kentucky Fried Chicken with him on the way home!

You probably won't realise, and no one will ever tell you, that you might need to soften some of your old values or adopt new ones when you transition. You need to work that out for yourself. The hope of this chapter is to get you thinking about your values in detail and asking the question whether they will serve you well moving forward or not.

A great framework that I think is useful for this process is an adaptation of a business model I came across while studying my MBA. It is called the *Three Box Solution* and was developed by Vijay Govindarajan (VG).

The model has a cool backstory that comes from Hindu cosmology and is centred around three gods: Vishnu; the preserver, Shiva; the destroyer, and Brahma; the creator.

In the Hindu universe, there is no beginning or end, and the constant cycle of life relies on balanced creation, preservation, and destruction. When applied to businesses this model allows leaders to look at which processes are no longer useful or productive and should be discontinued; which are fundamental to their current operation and productivity and should be sustained; and which are going to prepare them for their future and should be developed.

I reckon the same process can be applied to our values during the transition period out of military or first responder roles.

Call to action: Apply the Three Box Solution to your values.

Start with the list of your values created in Chapter 3 and add any other specific organisational values that may still be ingrained into you from your previous role (maybe look up the organisational values of your old organisation if you don't know them specifically).

Now, think ahead to the person you want to evolve into to thrive post-transition and what values you might need to develop to get there. This is going to be imperfect, as it's impossible to predict with certainty where you're headed, but just do your best. The goal is to be considering it.

Now place the individual values from your list into one of the three boxes in the table below.

Values that no longer serve you and should be softened or let go	Current values that will serve you well post-transition and should be kept	Values you think you need to develop or strengthen to thrive post-transition

12. Show me your friends and I'll show you your future

I've never been one to keep in touch with my ex-girlfriends. I just never saw the point. There was always a good reason why we had broken up in the first place (sometimes my own poor judgement and wrongdoing), but it was more than that. The one occasion when I did try to stay in close touch with an ex was after she had dumped me, and it left me in an odd sort of limbo. We were no longer together, yet for a period of months afterwards I was struggling to adjust to that fact. The times when I did see her were awkward and I eventually realised that it was well and truly over and the best thing I could do for my own mental health was to sever ties with her and move on. It was tough, but necessary.

Now admittedly I was young at the time, and we weren't married and didn't have kids together. Thankfully my one go at marriage is still going strong, so I haven't faced the pain of trying to negotiate the situation where a serious relationship has broken down with the need to maintain the relationship with an ex because of kids. I can only imagine the complexity of that situation, but I also imagine that some of the principles of this chapter might apply.

If you stay overly engaged in your former relationship despite it being over, it makes it very difficult to meaningfully move forward with any new intimate relationship. I see transition out of the military or a first responder role as a similar situation. You have in effect broken up with your tribe and yet you are likely to still identify as part of that in-group.

Everyone is different, but if you fail to start to soften these links back to your old tribe it will make it near impossible to solve your identity crisis (you may not even realise that you have one) and explore new social relationships that might eventually lead to integration into new in-groups. You will get left in the same limbo that I found myself in after I was dumped, where I still felt like I was in the old relationship, when clearly, I wasn't. During that period the last thing on my mind was trying to meet new girls and perhaps build a new relationship. In effect, it was like a micro identity crisis. The part of me that identified as being in a relationship needed time to adjust to the new situation and then eventually evolve to identifying as being single again, before being at the stage of looking for another potential relationship.

American businessman Dan Pena is quoted as saying "show me your friends and I'll show you your future", which applies here.

We all tend to gravitate towards people who we share interests and values with. It's likely that to some degree this contributes to people joining the military or first responder organisations in the first place. They have a certain set of values and beliefs that draw them towards that line of work, and they then find themselves surrounded by others with similar values, beliefs, and interests.

For the reasons discussed in this book, that all gets amplified throughout their training and subsequent careers to often reach the point of identity-fused in-group affiliation. Over time, it can also lead to what the psychologists call *cultural myopia*, being the situation where your in-group is so focused on a particular set of values and beliefs that they become metaphorically myopic (short sighted) and unable to see different points of view.

In extreme situations this cause some of the negative aspects of *groupthink*[21], but for the most part it is a positive force that bonds the group together. It does however become a problem on transition out of the former in-group and can fuel the loneliness felt when back in the broader community.

An overwhelming temptation can be to gravitate back towards socialising with members of your former tribe, but you need to accept that you are no longer one of them. That doesn't mean you can't hang out with your old work buddies, but it does mean that you need to soften the part of you that identifies with being one of them and start identifying as being a *former* one of them. If you continue to exclusively

---

[21] Some of the negative aspects of groupthink include collective rationalisation of inappropriate actions, toxic stereotyping of out-groups, an illusion of invulnerability, and direct pressure on dissenters within the group.

hang out with your former tribe members, then it becomes a case of show me your friends and I'll show you your past.

There's another similar saying that is attributed to motivational speaker Jim Rohn that suggests *you're the average of the five people that you spend the most time with*. Now, this concept is not without its critics, but I think the principle is useful to this discussion. If the five people you are hanging around with most post-transition are your former work mates who are still in the job, then it will be very difficult to form a positive new identity and move forward in life. You'll get stuck in an identity no-man's-land.

I'm not suggesting that you need to cut ties with all of your former work mates and start fresh with a new group of five people to surround yourself with. At first, you will likely crave the company of your former tribe and during transition it can be comforting to hang out with them and stay connected. You might have some shared interests and hobbies outside of work that you can still do with them. Over time though, you must begin to consciously acknowledge that you have left their tribe and invest in relationships that support your new identity. It is only in doing this that you will ever be able to build friendships that are aligned with your future rather than your past.

During my transition out of the army, I found it useful to seek out veterans who had transitioned prior to me and successfully reintegrated back into civilian life. In a way, they represented the best of both worlds in that I could relate to them on the level of our shared military past and, having done it themselves, they could also serve as mentors to help me negotiate my reintegration into civilian life.

Call to action: Do your friends represent your future or your past?

List the people you spend most of your time with and categorise them as to whether they represent your past, future, or both (in the instance of former work mates who you share a future focused relationship with).

Are there any in your top five who your future is aligned with? If not, perhaps start by investing just a little more time with at least one person who is not a member of your former tribe and go from there. Open your mind to different points of view that they may hold and start to overcome any cultural myopia that you may have developed in your former role.

Friend name	Past	Future	Both

13. Civilians will not find you funny

Humour, and particularly dark humour, is a fantastic way to diffuse stressful situations and make a little light of traumatic events. Generally, only other members of your tribe, or those with cultures closely aligned, will find dark humour funny and taken out of context by those not indoctrinated into a military or first responder culture it can be perceived as terribly inappropriate and insensitive. In this day and age of sensitivity and political correctness, coupled with the ever-increasing capture of imagery with smartphones, CCTV, and body-worn cameras, dark humour must be used with situational awareness and caution. However, the right joke to the right audience at the right time can be a brilliant tool.

Let me give you an example from a distant time in a faraway place.

This story takes place in a rudimentary surgical facility in a regional area of a warzone. Our element had been conducting a targeting operation and just before making entry into a designated compound a large explosion erupted from within.

After rendering the scene safe and clearing the compound, we found a horribly injured enemy fighter, who we medically stabilised and evacuated to a surgical facility. He had been arming an Improvised Explosive Device to kill and maim members of our element, and it had initiated in the process resulting in what was colloquially known as an *own goal*.

By the look of the fighter, he couldn't have been more than 17 years of age, and the pattern of his injuries suggested that he had been crouched over the device when it initiated. He had lost a foot and a hand, and his lower limbs and genitals were badly damaged. As his eyes had been focused on the device when it went off, he had lost both of those also, in among other serious facial injuries.

It was a truly horrific scene, and there were significantly mixed emotions in the resuscitation room. On one hand the fighter had clear intent on killing our task group members. On the other hand, he was either a young man fighting for a cause that he believed to be right, or he had been pressured by the enemy to join the fight with non-compliance likely having lethal consequences for himself and possibly his family.

It was in this context that one of the surgeons on the treating team drew our detailed attention to the state of the enemy's genitals. His scrotum had been badly lacerated in multiple areas and his testicles were partially protruding from both sides. The dark humour comment from the surgeon diffused the situation beautifully.

"Looks like Admiral Ackbar!" the surgeon exclaimed.

For those readers unfamiliar with the Star Wars character Admiral Ackbar, I encourage you to pause reading here and google an image of him. Naturally the surgeon's comments were followed by a chorus of "IT'S A TRAP!" from all in attendance, being Ackbar's most famous (perhaps only?) line in the Star Wars movies.

Now, I realise the insensitivity of that comment in absolute terms, however if you're reading this book then you've probably used dark humour to diffuse tense situations and can appreciate the joke here. For us at the time it served as the perfect tool to ease the tension of the moment and looking back on that scene in my mind's eye now, over a decade later, the humour is my enduring memory, not the sadness of the situation. It is however a story that I know not to share in the presence of those outside of the military and first responder communities and I can proudly say that I've never cracked it out at dinner parties with my wife's friends.

The use of humour

Humour is yet another social concept that most of us never really stop to think deeply about. We know what is funny to us and most will have some awareness that not everyone finds the same things funny and that a joke that makes one person laugh might be deeply offensive to another.

In military and first responder roles, humour is very culturally specific and gets used in unique ways when compared to its use in broader society.

For example, to get a chuckle out of the Admiral Ackbar joke mentioned above, you need to have a certain degree of desensitisation to the traumatic nature of the context and be able to temporarily look past the tragedy of the young man being permanently disabled by the explosion. Someone without this desensitisation would likely fixate on the magnitude of the man's injuries and then find the *attempt* at humour in the context deeply offensive. For that person, the joke would miss its mark completely.

Humour as a construct has been extensively studied and many theories exist. Three key theories[22] are:

- **Relief theory** – humour is used to reduce anxiety, fear, or suffering. Basically, it's used as a defence mechanism to help take your mind away from the harsh reality you're facing. This is the textbook *if I don't laugh, I'll cry* situation.

- **Incongruity theory** – Humour is derived from an incongruence, or a lack of fit, between the humour object and the context that it exists within. Basically, the humour exists in the space between the object and the context.

- **Superiority theory** – humour is used as a social tool to position oneself, or one's group, in relation to another. Most often, the joke will be at the expense of another individual or group to position the joke maker as superior.

[22] John C. Meyer, Humor as a Double-Edged Sword: Four Functions of Humor in Communication, *Communication Theory*, Volume 10, Issue 3, 1 August 2000, Pages 310–331

In the Admiral Ackbar joke, a degree of relief theory and incongruity theory are at play. The joke was used to diffuse the trauma of the situation and was funny due to the incongruence between a badly damaged body part and its uncanny resemblance to a Star Wars character.

There's no issue per se with the use of either of these forms of humour, but what makes the joke controversial is the extreme nature of the circumstances under which it was made.

Research suggests that dark humour translates well across the boundaries of different first responder groups, for instance what a paramedic finds funny will probably also make a police officer laugh[23]. But while this might extend to include other groups with similar experiences, such as military, firefighters, and correctional officers, care needs to be taken with using this sort of dark humour in the presence of those outside of military and first response roles. Those without the same desensitisation are unlikely to find dark humour funny and may even be offended (or traumatised) by something that you and your former tribe might think is hilarious.

Looping back to the theories of humour, superiority fits into the previously discussed aspects of social identity theory that are at play in military and first responder or-ganisations. The tendency to joke in a derogatory nature

---

[23] Charman, S.J. (2013). Sharing a laugh: The role of humour in relationships between police officers and ambulance staff. *International Journal of Sociology and Social Policy*, 33, 152-166.

towards out-groups can serve to strengthen in-group cohesion and esprit de corps. While a degree of this can be productive, taken to extremes it can become toxic.

When we look at humour in the context of hierarchical rank structures, such as those found in the military and first responder organisations, it reveals another interesting use of the construct. Humour can be used as a way of conveying information up the chain of command in the form of a joke where, if the information were otherwise delivered in a serious way, it would be considered insubordinate.

Sarcasm, being the practice of saying one thing and meaning the opposite, is often used for these means. Those in leadership roles who are tuned in to this practice can read between the lines to interpret the information being conveyed and act on it accordingly. This subtle practice relies on an established relationship, and the use of sarcasm in less established relationships is likely to create the perception of conflict.

Gaining insight into your humour style can be a useful thing to do in transition and there's a questionnaire for exactly this, aptly named the Humor Styles Questionnaire (HSQ). The HSQ measures four humour styles:

Affiliative Humour

People high on affiliative humour enjoy sharing humour with other people. They like to tell jokes that include others, without being at the expense of others. They don't take themselves too seriously and can make jokes about their own mistakes.

Research suggests that those who score highly on affiliative humour are generally cheerful, outgoing, friendly, and tend to have good relationships with others.

Self-enhancing Humour

People high on self-enhancing humour tend to always look on the funny side of life and can maintain this outlook even in times of stress and adversity. Even when they're alone, they are amused by life's absurdities and can have a laugh.

Research shows that those high in self-enhancing humour tend to be emotionally well adjusted, cope well with stress, are optimistic, and don't easily become discouraged, anxious, or depressed.

Aggressive Humour

People high on aggressive humour tend to use humour to tease, put down, or manipulate other people. Although they may be very witty, their humour is often laced with ridicule or sarcasm, and they are often not concerned if their humour is hurtful to others, including the use of sexist or racist jokes.

Those high on aggressive humour tend to make fun of others to enhance their own self-esteem. Research suggests they are often aggressive and insensitive to others, and that their use of aggressive humour doesn't lead to any improved levels of self-esteem or emotional wellbeing.

Self-defeating Humour

People high in self-defeating humour, while often funny, tend to go too far in making jokes at their own expense and putting themselves down in an amusing way. They are generally happy to be the butt of jokes with a view to making others accept them, however research suggests that they are often low on self-esteem and dissatisfied with their relationships. They tend to use humour to hide their true emotions, putting on a happy face to the outside world while being unhappy inside.

If you're anything like me, you will have probably developed a healthy dose of aggressive humour during your time with the military or first responder organisation, and you'll favour dark humour delivered in a sarcastic manner! You can probably gather by now that this isn't the most productive humour style to move forward with post-transition.

In the years that followed my transition from the army I started to tune into my humour style and realise clearly that it was poorly suited to my professional roles. I became aware of my tendency to interrupt work meetings with jokes (that weren't always well received) and my constant use of sarcasm and aggressive humour.

What really drilled it home to me was seeing my humour style reflected back at me in my sons' jokes as they started to develop their own senses of humour based on me as a role model. Since that time, I've become far more aware of my humour style and aimed to use more affiliative and self-enhancing humour, especially in front of my kids. I do, however, still love a bit of dark humour here and there in the appropriate circumstances and company!

Call to action: What is your humour style?

Do the Humor Styles Questionnaire (which at the time of writing is available free online at www.humorstyles.com). Place your scores in the following table:

Humour Style	%ile
Affiliative Humour	
Self-Enhancing Humour	
Aggressive Humour	
Self-Defeating Humour	

Do you think your results show the best use of humour to move forward with post-transition?

If not, try to tune in to your use of humour and see if you can start to crack some more affiliative and self-enhancing jokes, and maybe drop a little of the sarcasm and aggressive humour.

One person who will give you a no bullshit appraisal of how funny you are is a psychologist. Let's chat about the other benefits of seeing one in the next chapter.

14. You can stop lying to the psych (and start seeing one by choice!)

I have never been a police officer; however, I have had a lot to do with police and police psychologists over the years and feel I have gained an insight into why the average copper is suspicious of psychologists.

If I might, I'd like to share my theory.

While I've singled out police officers in this example, the same theory is almost definitely applicable to the broader military and first responder communities.

Before we get into why cops are sus on psychologists, I want to deviate and have a look at use of force, in particular the extreme end of the spectrum, being the use of lethal force.

Let's consider the example of a police officer arriving on a scene where a perpetrator has a gun and is firing rounds into a crowd. Upon arrival of the police, the perp turns their attention to them and starts firing well-aimed shots at the cops. Ask the average police officer how they would react to this scenario, and I imagine the vast majority, if not all, would reply with *shoot back!*

In this setting the use of lethal force is clearly justified. The police officer's life, as well as the lives of innocent crowd members, is at risk and as such the police officer has a professional obligation to resolve the situation. They are empowered by law to employ lethal force and as much as they may not want to harm another human, it is the ugly task that society requires them to do under appropriate circumstances and it is why police in most jurisdictions carry firearms.

Jumping back now to police-psychologist interactions, from my experience with the two groups, most interactions between them seem to fall into two categories.

The first is the mandated psychological screens after critical incidents, where it is anecdotally commonplace for the cop to tell the psychologist what they want to hear to tick the boxes and make it go away so they can get on with policing.

The second category of interaction then usually doesn't occur until the psychological wheels are coming off and the police officer's trauma bucket has filled and is flowing over. By this stage it is no longer possible for the cop to hide the fact that they are experiencing psychological issues and they find themselves in front of a psychologist.

It is often only at this point that the police officer is willing to disclose what has been going on for the first time. The cat is out of the bag anyway and it can no longer be hidden. Unfortunately for the psychologist this is generally the first they are hearing of the issue, when things are at crisis point and the police officer is suffering from a significant acute psychological injury.

Just like a cop needing to escalate immediately to lethal force when turning up to the scene where a perp is spraying bullets everywhere, the psychologist has an obligation to act appropriately when an acutely unwell police officer ends up in their office. This may well involve a recommendation to the chain of command that the officer have their badge and gun taken from them for a period until they are in a psychologically better place and thinking more clearly again.

Just like the cop not wanting to take a life, the psych doesn't want to sideline the cop, but both groups shoulder the duty of care responsibility to do what they are professionally obliged to do, and what is safe and right.

The result is a misconception that the psychologist should be feared, wrongfully assuming that they *want* to take a cop's badge and gun. This serves to perpetuate the stigma of psychologists that is common among not only police, but the broader military and first responder communities.

Let's now back up and look at the situation where a police officer turns up to a scene where a perpetrator with a gun is starting to escalate but hasn't yet shot a single round.

In that setting the cop has not yet had their hand forced to shoot back immediately and has other options to potentially resolve the situation without the use of lethal force. It may be that a skilled negotiation could deescalate the situation, or perhaps the use of a less-than-lethal option such as Taser, chemical incapacitant, or physical restraint could be employed to neutralise the perp and render the scene safe.

The exact same principles can be applied to the cop-psychologist interaction.

If the police officer ends up in the psychologist's office *before* things have hit crisis point, the psych has options available to them to get the cop back on track without having to temporarily take their badge and gun (their metaphoric use of lethal force).

The key is to deal with the situation before it gets to crisis point, and the onus is on the individual to recognise that they are having issues, and then have the insight and vulnerability to seek professional help before they spiral downward to the point where the psychologist has no other safe option than to sideline them from their role.

Why military members and first responders fear psychologists

So, why exactly is it that military members and first responders often don't seek psychological support before the wheels have come off it? There are some great studies into exactly this, with my favourite being that of Burns & Buchanan (2020) who asked the question of a large cohort of Canadian police officers in their article *Factors that influence the decision to seek help in a police population*[24].

---

[24] Burns C, Buchanan M. Factors that Influence the Decision to Seek Help in a Police Population. Int J Environ Res Public Health. 2020 Sep 21;17(18):6891.

Three of the key reasons they cite will probably come as no surprise to anyone reading:

1. The stigma of being perceived as weak or incompetent
2. Concerns about being labelled unfit for duty
3. Worry that accessing psychological support will impact future career advancement

These are all legitimate concerns for serving military members or first responders and unfortunately remain barriers to seeking psychological support.

Somewhat predictably, the study also found that police interviewed didn't hold the same degree of stigma against physical injuries as they did towards mental health issues and were more accepting of an acute stress reaction following major incidents, but less accepting of long-term cumulative stress issues.

Having spent their career solidifying these views on mental health issues and support, this attitude towards mental health support becomes part of the military or first responder's identity and gets counterproductively carried into transition out of the role. This is a perception that needs to be challenged during the transition process and put into the *values that no longer serve you and should be softened or let go* box from Chapter 11.

When we look at the three key reasons why police didn't seek psychological support listed above, two of them are often no longer relevant post-transition, those being; labelled unfit for duty, and impact on career advancement (accepting that a mental health diagnosis might have implications on future career prospects in some cases).

All psychological diagnoses aside, research tells us that the majority of transitioning members will experience significant stress during the period (transition stress) and having a mental health specialist in your corner during transition is highly recommended.

Looking at the situation through the lens of the army special operations elements I used to work with, we would take a range of different specialists into the field with us. As a doctor I was one of them. Key among the others in operational environments where the IED threat was high were our special operations engineers. Makes sense, right? If you have a specialist problem, then you want a specialist to resolve it. It's no different when optimising your mental health during transition, you want someone on your team with the right training and experience to help you solve complex problems.

Other perceptions that I've commonly heard as barriers to seeking psychological support are: *what would they know?, they haven't done the job? Or they don't know me.*

Those things may be true, and certainly a culturally-informed psychologist is preferable to one who has no understanding of the unique stressors of military or first response work, however these questions that often serve as barriers can equally be viewed as strengths.

The fact that the psychologist may not have an intimate knowledge of the member, or their former role, means that they will have no established preconceived ideas as to what to expect and no significant emotional attachment that could otherwise potentially cloud their assessment and advice. This might serve to improve their ability to maintain the necessary professional distance to see the situation objectively and provide unbiased support and advice.

The real power of psychologists and other mental health professionals however is that they have the evidence-based tools to help deal with the stress of transition and start to process any accumulated psychological burden that may not have been addressed during service. Furthermore, they are a great sounding board during the period of identity crisis that occurs during the transition period.

Your former tribe members and family and friends are also great sources of support during this period (more on that in Chapter 18) but it's unlikely that any of them will have the professional tools to help in an evidence-based fashion. Asking them to help you work through psychological issues is like handing a metal detector and specialist engineer tools to an untrained operator and asking them to find and diffuse an IED. In that situation, it's toss a coin whether they find and diffuse the device, or whether things blow up!

I challenge you to think of psychologists and counsellors as like being *mechanics for your mind*.

You don't want to wait for your car to break down to get it towed to a mechanic to be fixed. If you get it serviced and tuned up regularly, it's far less likely to break down in the first place. The same is true for your mental health. If you're getting a mental tune up regularly from a psychologist or counsellor, then you're far less likely to have your mental machinery break down.

Call to action: Challenge your perception of psychologists and counsellors.

The following questions are taken from a tool known as the *attitude toward seeking professional psychological help short-scale form*[25] *(ATSPPH-SF)*. Have a look at them and consider whether you would disagree, partially disagree, partially agree, or agree.

1. If I believed I was having a mental breakdown, my first inclination would be to get professional attention.

2. The idea of talking about problems with a psychologist strikes me as a poor way to get rid of emotional conflicts.

3. If I were experiencing a serious emotional crisis at this point in my life, I would be confident that I could find relief in psychotherapy.

4. There is something to admire about a person who copes with conflicts and fears without going for professional help.

5. I would want to get psychological help if I was worried or upset for a long period of time.

---

[25] Fischer, E. H., and Farina, A. (1995). Attitudes toward seeking professional psychological help: a shortened form and considerations for research. *J. Coll. Stud. Dev.* 36, 368–373.

6. I might want to have psychological counselling in the future.

7. A person with an emotional problem is not likely to solve it alone; he or she is likely to solve it with professional help.

8. Considering the time and expense involved in psychotherapy, it would have little value for a person like me.

9. A person should work out his or her own problems; getting psychological counselling would be a last resort.

10. Personal and emotional troubles, like many things, tend to work out by themselves.

If you're like most military and first responders, you probably disagree with statements 1,3,5,6, and 7, and agree with 2,4,8,9, and 10!

If so, that's not surprising. Military and first responder cultures favour stoicism, keeping problems to yourself, and the attitude of getting on with it despite adversity. However, these values might be ones that you need to soften after transition (remember Chapter 11!) to move forward as the best version of yourself.

One final point of consideration is what you would say to a struggling former teammate?

Would you advise them to suck it up and struggle on alone, or would you encourage them to see a psychologist or counsellor?

I bet that most people reading would choose the latter, so why don't we apply that same principle to ourselves?

15. Don't expect anyone to care that you served.

The first job that I had after transition from the army was as a fly-in, fly-out, doctor on a mine site. As I established myself in that role, it became clear pretty quickly that aside from a few people here and there, no one gave two shits about my military service.

This came as a bit of a blow to my ego for sure and with hindsight I had probably left the army a little fuller of my own self-importance that I was objectively entitled to be. I had naively expected that a degree of the prestige and status that I had earned in the army might come with me on transition and into my new role.

Wrong!

It took me a little while to realise the harsh truth of the situation; that I was the new guy and I needed to earn my stripes and prove myself in my new work role before I would be afforded any status and prestige in that organisation.

Once I had checked my ego, I started to come to peace with the fact that much of broader society really has no idea

what service in the military or a first response organisation entails and often they don't care. I don't mean that in
a derogatory way, I simply mean that they have been busy
establishing themselves in their own professional and social
in-groups and have had no cause to learn or understand
what is involved in military or first responder work and
therefore have no reason to hold it in any sort of esteem.

Even when people did show appreciation for my military
service, I still needed to establish my credibility in my new
work role.

In that setting it was a case of *thank you for your service,
now prove yourself.*

I firmly believe that this is exactly as it should be and
while it's always nice to have someone acknowledge the
unique sacrifices of military or first responder work, there
should be no expectation of preferential treatment or entitlement in a new work environment. If you can use your
previous service to get a foot in the door somewhere, then
great – go for it, but then you need to knuckle down and use
the same grit that you used in your former role to establish
yourself in your new one.

At the time when I was getting my ego bruised on the
mine site and coming to the realisation that I needed to start
again in building credibility, I came to reflect on the story of
a soldier who I had formerly served with.

This bloke had been a professional football player before
enlisting in the army and ending up at the infantry unit I
was serving with at the time. There were some big footy fans

at the unit, and this earned him a certain degree of status among the troops when he turned up, but I never once saw him try to use it to his advantage. If anything, he was quickly dismissive of any mention of his former football career and achievements. He simply put his head down and concentrated on his soldiering.

Ultimately, from a military perspective, his previous professional sporting accomplishments meant very little, he needed to prove himself in this new environment. And prove himself he did. He quickly progressed to being one of the best soldiers in his platoon, qualified for reconnaissance platoon, and then ultimately successfully completed SAS selection and moved into special operations.

In my opinion he epitomised the point that no matter how accomplished you may have been in your former role you shouldn't expect any of your former prestige to transition with you. You need to take the ego hit, then get busy with proving yourself in your new role.

Generativity versus Stagnation

At the time when I discharged from the army, I was fast approaching my 40s and from a psychological perspective was entering the life stage that Erikson (remember him from Chapter 3?) referred to as *Generativity versus Stagnation*.

Erikson proposes that as we enter our middle age, we begin to reflect on our life experiences and accomplishments and often feel a desire to give back to society. For parents this can take the form of investment in their kids, and professionally it can be the teaching and mentoring of younger generations coming through the workplace.

For me, I had started to do that prior to my transition as an instructor in the special operations medical community, both domestically and internationally. I had established a degree of experience in tactical medicine, and I found using that to train the new generation of medics and doctors coming into special operations hugely rewarding. I felt as though I was leaving a positive legacy from my time in the army.

I had been experiencing what Erikson called *generativity* and while I remained established in my military career things were rosy in this department. The obvious problem occurred when I discharged and lost access to the activities that were fuelling this sense of generativity.

The opposite of generativity in Erikson's model is *stagnation*, being feelings of not contributing to society in a meaningful or fulfilling fashion. Stagnation can lead to feelings of unfulfillment, a sense of purposelessness, apathy, and a struggle to find meaning and direction in life.

This definitely captures how I felt in my first job post-transition out of the army. Slowly but surely however, I started to move the needle back in the direction of generativity.

Initially, that came from running trauma management training for the paramedics on the mine site. Then, over time, I started my own tactical medical training company and subsequently bought into a larger existing company, allowing me to further achieve generativity by using my skills to train those who might need them.

As I moved from the mine site job to the role at a small hospital, I was then able to further this sense of contribution via not only feeling a greater sense of purpose for the work I was doing in the emergency department, but also helping to train the junior doctors and nurses in the hospital. All of this contributed to rebuilding the psychological layers of my Maslow's Hierarchy.

Erikson proposes that the generativity versus stagnation stage lasts from the ages of around 40-65. For those who transition out of the military or first responder roles in this age range, it's essential to find activities to create a sense of generativity.

If you've transitioned due to medical or psychological injury, it's still equally important to find activities that allow generativity to be achieved and to avoid stagnation. This might be a contribution to a veteran's group or Returned Services League for military members, or the equivalent for other emergency response groups.

The activities used to achieve generativity needn't necessarily be aligned with your former skills, the contribution could be broader, such as volunteering at a local school, involvement in local government, sporting teams, or even neighbourhood organisations. Equally, if you have kids, the contribution could be closer to home through an increased investment of time with your kids.

The *what* doesn't matter so much, it's the *why*; that being a sense of contribution to society.

Call to action: How are you contributing to society?

List your current contributions that add to a sense of generativity (don't worry if there aren't any at this stage – that's what this call to action is all about!)	
List the key skills you have that might be of value to a younger generation, or the community more broadly (use the list of professional qualifications and skills from Chapter 3 as a start)	
Brainstorm some groups you might be interested in and able to contribute to. Think widely here and not just of those aligned with your former profession. Examples might include: • Schools • Cubs/ Scouts/Girl Guides • Local sporting teams • Local council • Body corporates	

16. You are not broken, you are more complete

I wrote about this same topic towards the end of my book *The Combat Doctor*. For years following my discharge from the army I felt like I had somehow been broken by my service. That perhaps a part of me had died on the battlefields of Afghanistan. It took me a few years into my transition to start thinking of things differently, to reframe what I was experiencing and start to view myself as not broken, but more complete.

A couple of frameworks that helped with this reframing were the concept of our *inner monster* described by contemporary psychologist and public intellectual Jordan Peterson, and the concept that I interpret Peterson's monster to be based on, being our *shadow* as described by the 20th century psychiatrist Carl Jung (remember him from the loneliness quote in Chapter 10?).

Starting with Jung, he proposed that the human *psyche* is comprised of "…the totality of all psychic processes, conscious as well as unconscious"[26]. A diagrammatic representation of Jung's psyche can be found at Figure 11.

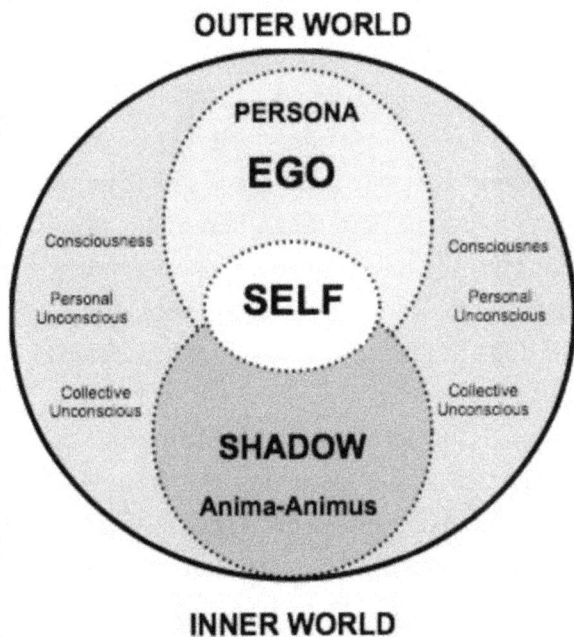

Figure 11. Jung's construct of the psyche (image source: www.thebtseffect.com)

On the conscious side of the model are our *Persona* and the *Ego*.

The persona comes about as a means of adapting to one's environment. It's a social mask that we wear to fit into society.

---

[26] Jung, CG. 1971. *The collected works of CG Jung, Volume 6*, Princeton University Press, NJ.

The ego is our conscious awareness of existing and a continuous sense of personal identity.

Jung used the analogy of consciousness as being like an eye, only a limited number of things can be held in vision at the one time and the rest is either in the periphery or remains not seen or focused on.

On the *personal unconscious* (often denied or repressed) side of the model are our *shadow* and *anima* or *animus*.

The shadow is the part of us where all the things that we either don't want to know, or do not like, exist. It is the parts of us that are often opposite to our persona; the parts that we know don't fit the societal norms that we're expected to abide by.

Jung used the terms anima and animus to describe the contrasexual archetype, being the feminine side of a masculine person (anima – aspects such as empathy, related-ness, and nurturance) and the masculine side of a feminine person (animus – aspects such as aggression, autonomy, and separateness).

The *Self* represents the whole of the psyche and exists at the intersection of the individual's conscious (persona and ego) and unconscious (shadow and anima/animus) selves.

Outside of the personal unconscious exists the *collective unconscious*.

Jung theorised that we are all born hardwired with a blueprint of *how* to be a human, including instincts and archetypes: ancient primal symbols that are seen replicated across cultures and religions worldwide. These include, amongst others, the archetypical mother figure (The Great Mother) and profound elders as sources of knowledge (Wise Old Man). The collective unconscious helps us to make sense of our world and experiences.

Through their exposures and occupational desensitisation, military members and first responders may have formed perspectives on subjects such as death, human suffering, humour, empathy, and compassion, that differ from the norms of broader society's collective unconscious. This can compound the feelings of alienation and isolation felt by individuals in transition as they attempt to reintegrate into a society that views these subjects very differently.

Jung referred to the search for wholeness in our psyche as *individuation*. This requires the acknowledgement of our unconscious shadow and anima/animus and integration of them into our conscious self. Jung proposes that this process will create conflict and it is the resolution of this conflict that moves us towards being more complete.

Jung referred to the process of acknowledging our shadow as *shadow work*, and on it he comments:

> "This confrontation is the first test of courage on the inner way, a test sufficient to frighten off most people, for the meeting with ourselves belongs to the more unpleasant things that can be avoided so long as we can project everything negative into the environment. But if we are able to see our own shadow and can bear knowing about it, then a small part of the problem has already been solved: we have at least

brought up the personal unconscious. The shadow is a living part of the personality and therefore wants to live with it in some form. It cannot be argued out of existence or rationalized into harmlessness. This problem is exceedingly difficult, because it not only challenges the whole man, but reminds him at the same time of his helplessness and ineffectuality."[27]

Following on from Jung and elaborating on his work is the Jungian psychoanalyst Dr Murray Stein. On the topic of shadow work, Stein offers:

"The problem of integrating the shadow is a moral and psychological problem of the most thorny sort. If a person completely shuns the shadow, life is proper but it is terribly incomplete. By opening up to shadow experience, however, a person becomes tainted with immorality but attains a greater degree of wholeness."[28]

When we consider Jordan Peterson's concept of the *inner monster*, it aligns nicely with Jung's shadow. And, like Jung, Peterson doesn't encourage us to ignore or repress it, but rather to *become* our inner monster and then tame it.

Peterson argues that if you're harmless you're simply weak and that true moral strength comes from becoming a formidable force and learning to control it. Peterson is

---

[27] Jung, CG. 1971. *The collected works of CG Jung, Volume 6*, Princeton University Press, NJ.

[28] Stein, M. 1999. *Jung's map of the soul*, Open Court, Illinois

quoted as saying:

> "And if you think tough men are dangerous, wait until you see what weak men are capable of".

Which echoes the Nietzsche quote:

> "…I have often laughed at the weaklings who thought themselves good because they had no claws".

Now, what does any of this have to do with transitioning military members or first responders? Let me explain.

For individuals to have entered the military or a first responder role in the first place, a certain set of things must have happened. They must have been born with a certain set of abilities and attributes and then been raised in an environment that shaped and influenced their choice of occupation.

There's a lot of different reasons why someone seeks out these kinds of professional roles, but one interesting suggestion is that people with more sociopathic/psychopathic traits can tend to gravitate towards joining the military or becoming a first responder.

Sociopathy and Psychopathy in military and first responders

When we think of sociopaths or psychopaths (often the terms are used interchangeably), we generally consider them to be bad people, and for the most part that is accurate. There are however some sociopathic/psychopathic personality traits that can prove quite protective, especially in unique roles such as military and first response. These traits include fearlessness, boldness (diminished fear reactivity), sensation seeking, and willingness to take risks.

It can be appreciated that these attributes might come in very handy in certain situations that a military member or first responder might find themselves in. Recent research in this area found that first responders surveyed scored significantly higher on measures of psychopathy, fearlessness, and boldness, than a control group of civilians[29]. The first responders also scored more highly in heroism and altruism, leading the researchers to propose that psychopathy and heroism might be two sides of the same coin in the first responder population.

Another trait associated with sociopathy/psychopathy is emotional coldness, or meanness.

While none of us want to be completely emotionally cold, in military and first responder work a degree of emotional distancing can be very protective.

Even if individuals have not been emotionally cold prior to joining the military or a first responder organisation, most will eventually become that way through regular exposures and desensitisation to human suffering.

This is one symptom in a condition that psychologists call *compassion fatigue*, which is characterised by emotional

---

[29] Patton CL, Smith SF, Lilienfeld SO. *Psychopathy and heroism in first responders: Traits cut from the same cloth?* Personal Disord. 2018 Jul;9(4):354-368.

and physical exhaustion leading to decreased empathy and compassion for others. Basically, it's when you run out of fucks to give!

Situational Psychopathy

Another relevant term that pops up in the scientific literature is *situational psychopathy*, being the adoption of psychopathic traits as an adaptive mechanism to a given situation.

Stein (the Jungian psychoanalyst referenced above) suggests that most people:

"...only reveal shadowy elements by accident, in dreams, or when pushed to extremes."[30]

Jung himself said:

"It is a frightening thought that man also has a shadow side to him, consisting not just of little weaknesses and foibles, but of a positively demonic dynamism. The individual seldom knows anything of this; to him, as an individual, it is incredible that he should ever in any circumstances go beyond himself".

Most people would like to deny that they are capable of horrible acts, and when discussing acts such as torture or murder, will honestly tell you that they wouldn't be capable of such things. They view people who commit these acts

---

[30] Stein, M. 1999. *Jung's map of the soul*, Open Court, Illinois

as being somehow fundamentally different to them. Both Jung and Stein would suggest otherwise, and propose that everyone is capable of doing horrible things under the right circumstances or *when pushed to extremes*.

A great point of discussion with those who deny their capacity to perform terrible acts is the hypothetical example of one of their children or loved ones being abused, and them being in a position of power to hurt or kill the abuser. In that hypothetical, most of these people would probably be able to imagine themselves inflicting violence on the perpetrator and perhaps even enjoying it, if only for a brief moment before their conscience kicked in. In that hypothetical, the person gets a quick and fictitious glimpse into their shadow, before quickly repressing the thought due to its incongruence with the collective unconscious.

But what if your occupation not only allows you, but on occasion encourages or incentivises you, to do the things that your shadow self might want to do? This can be the situation for some military members and first responders.

When I reflect on my time spent on Special Operations in Afghanistan, I can see that there were some very strange psychological factors at play. One of our task group's primary mission profiles was known as *kill/capture*. These missions were exactly what it says on the box: launching against designated enemies with the mission objective of doing one of those two things to them. Most of the targets we went after generally didn't want to be captured without a fight, so the kill option was often what resulted.

This was very much in the hit-zone for the shadow self. In that situation, not only was the use of force, up to and including lethal force, authorised when the rules of engagement were met, it was often required to achieve the mission objectives and therefore incentivised. The act of killing a designated target who didn't want to come without a fight was celebrated as it represented mission success. Through repeated exposures to these situations, military members can not only become supremely desensitised to killing and death, but in a strange Pavlovian way, start to positively reinforce it.

Looking again at Jung's diagrammatic model, situationally in warzones like Afghanistan, what should normally be a part of our unconscious shadow became very much part of our conscious Self. Over time in that abnormal role, it could then become not only part of our Ego, but also our Persona. The Special Operations Task Group that I deployed with was seen as, and saw ourselves as, soldiers who would launch on kill/capture missions and do what was required for mission success.

During my army career, I did four tours of Afghanistan in a four-year period. Some soldiers did ten or more tours. Whether or not any of us had sociopathic/psychopathic traits prior to joining the army (I suspect many did), the abnormal environment of targeting operations in Afghanistan certainly drove us towards them as an adaptive mechanism.

Measuring psychopathy

One clinical tool used to measure sociopathy/psychopathy, is the Levenson Self-Report Psychopathy Scale, which consists of 26 statements that are answered on a scale from *Disagree* through *Neutral* to *Agree*. Some questions are scored positively and some negatively. A snapshot of the statements from the tool is below:

- Success is based on survival of the fittest; I am not concerned about the losers
- I don't plan anything very far in advance
- I let others worry about higher values; my main concern is the bottom line
- Looking out for myself is the top priority
- I would be upset if my success came at someone else's expense
- I make a point of trying not to hurt others in pursuit of my goals
- I feel bad if my words or actions cause someone else to feel emotional pain

A similar scale used to assess aggression is aptly named *The Aggression Questionnaire*. It uses 29 questions to assess physical aggression, verbal aggression, anger, and hostility, using responses to statements including:

- Given enough provocation, I may hit another person
- If somebody hits me, I hit back
- I get into fights a little more than the average person
- If I have to resort to violence to protect my rights, I will

- I often find myself disagreeing with people
- I sometimes feel like a powder keg ready to explode

In the context of being deployed on operations in Afghanistan, my answers to these questionnaires put me firmly in the psychopathic and *anger management issues* categories on these scales. Living as my inner monster and my shadow self was the most adaptive version of myself for that environment, and over time it began to feel surprisingly normal and even good.

The problem would come when I returned to Australia and had to try to adjust back to a non-sociopathic version of myself. Part of me would crave the opportunity to go back to places like Afghanistan and become my shadow self again.

On discharge however, it became clear that there would be no further use for that version of myself. It was during this period, when I found myself surrounded by *normal* people again that it became apparent how *abnormal* I had become.

Reflecting on my time in Afghanistan left me feeling a significant amount of guilt and shame for some of the things I had been involved in, but moreso, guilt and shame for some of my experiences that I had no emotional reaction to whatsoever but knew that a *normal* person would be bothered by them. This left me feeling very much the psychopath until I eventually recognised that it was my shadow self, my inner monster, who had those experiences and as an adaptive mechanism had attached no emotion to them.

It had still been me, but just a different version of me that was required for the circumstances. Through doing Jung's shadow work, I eventually found peace and assurance in knowing that version of me is still within and can be called upon if the situation ever requires him in the future, however equally I know that he has no role in my day-to-day civilian life. I have met and become my inner monster and tamed him.

I appreciate that my example isn't representative of all military members and first responders. Some, in roles such as military, policing, and corrections, might be able to relate to the use of force example. With others however, I'm sure there is some degree of desensitisation and perhaps guilt for not feeling guilty associated with their experiences.

At a minimum, I suspect most will be suffering from a degree of compassion fatigue, involving emotional exhaustion leading to a blunting of empathy and compassion for others.

Returning to Jung's model, we find the anima/animus as the second component of our unconscious self and must strive to incorporate it as well when working towards individuation (the complete self).

Most military and first responder cultures are hypermasculine in nature to begin with, meaning that empathy and compassion are not generally aligned with the perceived priorities of the role. Couple that with a bit of compassion fatigue and these *feminine* traits can be lost completely in the military member or first responder.

While a blunting of empathy and compassion might be somewhat adaptive traits during an individual's career, after transitioning out of the role it is essential to rebuild them to thrive in society. And through deliberate effort it can be done.

Compassion Focussed Therapy

One leading researcher in the area of rebuilding empathy and compassion is Paul Gilbert, who coined the term *Compassion Focussed Therapy* (CFT)[31]

CFT is aimed at people who have high levels of shame and self-criticism and who might struggle to feel warmth and compassion towards themselves and others.

CFT is based on the relationships and balance between three types of emotion regulation systems that are hardwired into us from an evolutionary perspective:

1. **Threat and self-protection system:** which is designed to alert us to danger and direct our attention to threats in order to respond. Threat based emotions such as anger, anxiety, and disgust are associated with this system and it drives behaviours such as fight, flight, and freeze.

2. **Drive, seeking and acquisition focused system:** draws our attention to resources that might be of advantage to us, and is a positive system that creates drive to create and accomplish goals of significance to us.

---

[31] Gilbert P. *The origins and nature of compassion focused therapy.* Br J Clin Psychol. 2014 Mar;53(1):6-41.

3. **Contentment, soothing and affiliative system:** enables us to be at peace when we are no longer focused on threats or seeking out resources.

The goal of CFT is to move our focus away from the threat and self-protection system and more towards the compassion-based soothing system. This in turn will facilitate more of the positive drive towards goal creation and accomplishment.

This all starts with what Gilbert calls the *compassionate self*, which is optimised through attention in three areas[32]

1. Threat – developing a mindful and compassionate awareness of:
    o   Triggers in the body
    o   Feelings of anger, anxiety, shame, and disgust
    o   Rumination (going over negative thoughts in your mind)
    o   Self-criticism

2. Receiving / soothing
    o   Adaptive resilience building techniques
    o   Calming techniques such as breathing
    o   Grounding exercises
    o   Gratitude practice

3. Giving / doing
    o   Mindful acts of kindness

---

[32] Gilbert P. *The origins and nature of compassion focused therapy.* Br J Clin Psychol. 2014 Mar;53(1):6-41.

o   Practicing compassion to self and others
o   Formulating goals and driving behaviours
    towards them

A word of caution here – There's a lot of heavy stuff in this chapter with potential to stir some significant psychological demons. I highly recommend that anyone considering doing some shadow work or Compassion Focussed Therapy does so with an appropriately trained psychologist experienced in working with military and first responders. If you do attempt some of these techniques and find they're having negative psychological effects, stop immediately and seek help.

Adaptive resilience building techniques

As I negotiated my own transition, I reflected deeply on the factors that had made me so resilient when I was in the army and the factors that I had lost when I transitioned that left me vulnerable. That reflection led me to join forces with another two Special Operations veterans and write a book called *The Resilience Shield*[33].

In the book, we present resilience as a dynamic, multifactorial, and modifiable construct, which can be deliberately and proactively built in different areas of our lives. We call these areas the *Layers* of our Resilience Shield model, with the four readily modifiable layers being the:

---

[33] Pronk D, Pronk B, and Curtis T, 2021, *The Resilience Shield*, Macmillan Australia, Sydney.

- Mind Layer
- Body Layer
- Social Layer
- Professional Layer

Our model is evidence-based and backed by a research project in conjunction with the University of Western Australia that has enabled us to not only scientifically validate our model but also create a survey to quantify overall resilience, as well as score an individual's resilience in the four modifiable layers above.

Call To Action: Build your Resilience Shield

Start by getting across to www.resilienceshield.com and following the *assess your resilience* tab to find and complete our Resilience Survey. Write your scores in the boxes below.

	Score
Resilience Score	
Mind Layer	
Body Layer	
Social Layer	
Professional Layer	

Next thing to do is completely disregard your overall resilience score! This simply ranks your score on a Bell

Curve against the tens of thousands of other respondents and isn't useful for the purpose of building individual resilience. What is useful however is how you scored on the Mind, Body, Social, and Professional Layers. This lets you know where you are relatively strong and where your areas for improvement are.

Focus in on the areas where you scored the lowest and start to do some small, sustainable, interventions to improve those areas.

For a deep dive into the Resilience Shield Model and a comprehensive discussion of resilience building interventions across the layers, you can grab a copy of the book or check out our online courses available through www.resilienceshield.com

As a snapshot, here are some ideas to get you started across the Layers. The astute reader will recognise some repetition here from the cortisol regulating techniques mentioned in Chapter 7. That's not an error, regulating cortisol goes hand in hand with building resilience and these techniques are important enough to mention twice!

Resilience Shield Layer	Resilience Building Intervention
Mind Layer	• Try meditating – as little as 10 minutes a day is proven to make a huge difference. Guided meditation apps are a great place to start. • Practice grounding techniques such as taking a mindful moment to tune into your environment. Focus on five things you can see, four things you can feel, three things you can hear, two things you can smell, and one thing you can taste. • Have a go at Box Breathing to calm your nervous system. Breathe in deeply through your nose for four seconds, hold your breath for four seconds, breathe out for four seconds, and hold your breath for four seconds. Then repeat. • Practice Flow State activities – Remember those from Chapter 8? • Keep a journal to track how you feel and the key highs and lows of your transition journey. Focus here on what's going well and how you can improve the areas that aren't • Monitor your self-talk and cut it off quickly if you find it being negative or you're ruminating on bad memories from your past.

Body Layer	• Eat a balanced diet
	• Stay well hydrated
	• Do regular exercise – it doesn't matter what type.
	• Get out in the sunshine or daylight each morning, but be sun smart
	• Work on getting better sleep by:
	• Going to bed and getting up at a regular time
	• Reducing alcohol intake
	• Decreasing caffeine in the afternoon
	• Making your room as dark and quiet as you can
	• Keeping your room cool
	• Avoiding exercise or heavy meals close to bed time
	• Taking a warm bath a couple of hours before bed
	• Avoiding looking at screens or blocking the blue light from them in the hours before bed
Social Layer	• Make time (don't find it) to invest in building and maintaining key social relationships
	• Practice Active Listening, where you really listen to what people are saying rather than just waiting for your turn to talk. A great way to actively listen is to paraphrase back to a person what they have said to confirm your understanding of it
	• Schedule date nights with significant others

	• If you have pets, make time regularly to spend time with them (yes – pets count as part of your Social Layer) • Look for social or sporting groups you might like to join • Practice Psychological Transitions before social encounters, where you take a moment to check in with yourself and then ask yourself the following question "What's the best version of myself for this next interaction?"
Professional Layer	• Invest in your post-transition professional identity and try not to compare the role to your former one (remember Rosy Retrospection will probably cause you to remember things more positively than they were) • Look for the meaning and purpose in your post-transition role and stay focused on them • Do regular professional development activities to continually build your professional skills • When working, set up your workplace to minimise distractions and maximise productivity. Turn off notifications on your phone and email and only work on one thing at a time • Creating time limits for blocks of work is a great way to improve focus. One technique involves chunking work into 25 minute blocks, followed by a five-minute break before starting again.

	• Time Box your working day. Schedule your day into blocks of time dedicated to certain tasks, being sure to build in blocks to read and answer emails, to address short notice things that will inevitably pop up, and to rest.

17. What does not destroy me, makes me stronger

German philosopher Friedrich Nietzsche famously said, "Out of life's school of war: What does not destroy me, makes me stronger".

Some will be more familiar with the paraphrased version of the quote, "what doesn't kill me, makes me stronger", that holds the same meaning. What Nietzsche was recognising is the potential to grow following adversity.

We're all familiar with the concept of Post-Traumatic Stress Disorder (PTSD). It's very real, and in my opinion gets the rightful attention it deserves.

What I fear gets lost in the narrative on PTSD is that most people who experience significant life trauma and suffer from symptoms of post-traumatic stress recover back to their baseline level of function. The data varies widely based on the population studied, but certainly a vast majority (and up to 80% in some studies) make this recovery.

What is even less talked about are those who not only recover to their baseline level of function but transcend it and become a *better* version of themselves *because* of their trauma.

I consider myself to be one of these people and the psychologists refer to this concept as Post-Traumatic Growth (PTG).

Figure 12 illustrates the various outcomes after a significant traumatic event or the cumulative effect of complex trauma over time causing a mental health injury.

PTSD represents those who don't return to their baseline level of function, which can manifest in either succumbing to the symptoms or survival with impairment.

Return to baseline level of function following trauma can be considered as either recovery or resilience (the bouncing back definition of resilience).

Post-Traumatic Growth can be seen as transcending the point of recovery/resilience and thriving *because* of the traumatic exposure.

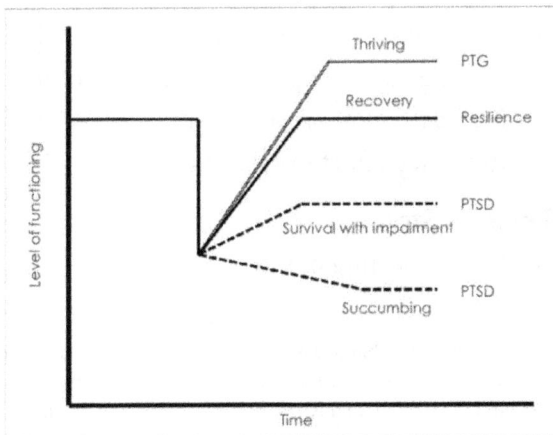

Figure 12. Outcomes after significant trauma (Jeon et al. 2015[34])

People who experience PTG can still have psychological distress related to their traumatic experiences. It's not
an either-or situation and the two can coexist. PTG simply
means that the individual has been able to find enough
positives out of their experiences to outweigh the negatives
and to facilitate personal growth.

The domains of Post Traumatic Growth

There are five domains of Post Traumatic Growth[35] as
follows:

- **New Possibilities**
  - o Developing new interests
  - o Establishing a new path in life
  - o Finding new meaning and purpose in life

- **Relating to Others**
  - o Greater sense of closeness with others
  - o Increased reliance on others in times of trouble
  - o Willingness to express emotions to others
  - o Increased compassion for others
  - o Increased effort in relationships

- **Personal Strength**
  - o Greater feeling of self-reliance

[34] Jeon, Sang Won & Han, Changsu & Choi, Joonho & Pae, Chi-Un & Chae,
Jeong-Ho & Ko, Young-Hoon & Yoon, Ho-Kyoung & Han, Changwoo.
(2015). *Posttraumatic Growth and Resilience: Assessment and Clinical
Implications.* Journal of Korean Neuropsychiatric Association. 54. 10.4306

[35] Tedeschi RG, Calhoun LG. *Trauma & transformation: growing in the
aftermath of suffering.* London: Sage Publications, 1995.

- o Increased ability to handle difficulties
- o Improved acceptance of life outcomes
- o New discovery of mental strength

- **Spiritual Change**
  - o Better understanding of spiritual matters
  - o Stronger religious (or spiritual) faith

- **Appreciation of Life**
  - o Changed priorities regarding what is important in life
  - o Greater appreciation of the value of one's own life
  - o Increased appreciation of each day

For years following my discharge from the army I carried a significant burden related to several key traumatic experiences in Afghanistan where I responded to teammates of mine and couldn't save them. I was very much in the realm of Post-Traumatic Stress, with regular intrusive thoughts of the events, bad dreams, and triggers including loud noises having the visceral reactions of making my heart race and my palms sweat.

For a period, the smell of raw pork would make me gag and occasionally vomit.

When I thought of my dead teammates, my over-whelming emotions were shame and guilt, and I made efforts to avoid anything that might trigger thoughts of my experiences (the maladaptive coping strategy of avoidance). Whenever possible, I stayed as busy as I could to distract myself from my thoughts (another maladaptive coping strategy – distraction).

Then one day, a few years after my discharge, it all changed. It was pretty much as sudden and dramatic as that, and I remember the experience vividly.

I was in my home gym when I began to consider how the soldiers we lost would have wanted me to feel about their deaths.

I considered the situation from my perspective, if I had been the bloke who was killed, and realised unquestionably that I wouldn't want those who tried their best to save me to be dwelling on it for years after the fact.

I would want them to be remembering me fondly, forgiving themselves for any perceived failure in trying to save me, and then living their very best lives in recognition that mine had been cut short.

I would want them to be the very best husbands they could be for those who were married, and the very best fathers they could be for those who had kids.

I realised in that moment that while I was physically present with my wife and kids, I was psychologically absent a lot of the time. I realised in that moment that I *owed* it to my dead teammates to do better.

That epiphany led to increased investment in my relationships with my wife and kids, and over time I began to experience a greater appreciation for life and everything that I had, as well as an increased sense of spirituality. I have never been a religious man, but more than ever I felt the sense of a greater power at play in the universe.

Over more time, my sense of gratitude for everything I have in my first-world life intensified and the ability to distil some of my experiences into books and presentations, delivered to those who I hoped might benefit from my lessons learned, further fuelled my post-traumatic growth.

The negative emotions attached to my experiences are still there if I go digging for them and that will never change. What I have achieved over the years, however, is the linking of more positive associations with the experiences, that I use as an ongoing drive to be the best version of myself that I can possibly be.

It's a work in progress and forever will be, but I can see now that… what didn't destroy me has made me stronger.

To borrow once more from the sage words of Carl Jung:
"I am not what happened to me, I am what I choose to become".

Call To action: Can you grow from your trauma?

A commonly used survey tool to assess for growth following trauma is the Post Traumatic Growth Inventory[36]. You can look it up online and complete it if you want your actual score, but as an idea of what factors are being assessed, it's based on ratings of 21 possible areas of growth and change following trauma. Have a look at the list below and consider

[36] Tedeschi RG, Calhoun LG (1996). "The posttraumatic growth inventory: Measuring the positive legacy of trauma". *Journal of Traumatic Stress.* 9 (3): 455–471.

whether you've experienced any of them because of your traumatic experiences. If so, focusing in on these positive outcomes is a great way to start reframing your trauma and seeing the silver lining to the cloud.

1. I changed my priorities about what is important in life
2. I have a greater appreciation for the value of my own life
3. I developed new interests
4. I have a greater feeling of self-reliance
5. I have a better understanding of spiritual matters
6. I more clearly see that I can count on people in times of trouble
7. I established a new path for my life
8. I have a greater sense of closeness with others
9. I am more willing to express my emotions
10. I know better that I can handle difficulties
11. I am able to do better things with my life
12. I am better able to accept the way things work out
13. I can better appreciate each day
14. New opportunities are available which wouldn't have been otherwise
15. I have more compassion for others
16. I put more effort into my relationships
17. I am more likely to try to change things which need changing
18. I have a stronger religious faith
19. I discovered that I'm stronger that I thought I was

20. I learned a great deal about how wonderful people are
21. I better accept needing others

18. You need a team to fight the battle with

One of the constants from my time with the military was that I was always surrounded by a team of people, especially when we were on missions in places like Afghanistan where it was likely we were going to run into trouble.

Before we even hit the ground, our intelligence teams were gathering and analysing all the information they could get their hands on to prepare us for what to expect.

Once we were out and about, every team member had their specialist roles, be it an assaulter, a breacher, a communicator, an engineer, a JTAC, a medic, the list goes on.

Having a diverse range of skills in the team allowed us to respond dynamically to challenges as they emerged and solve problems with expertise. We acknowledged that none of us had all the skills, and the authority at any given moment would go to the person on the ground who had the best skillset to match the immediate problem being encountered.

If that problem was the requirement for explosive entry to a compound, then the breachers took the lead. From there, the assaulters would take charge to prosecute the target. If an airstrike was required, all eyes were on the JTAC to guide the air support onto target. If we found an IED it was over to the engineers and if we sustained a casualty, then the medic would step up.

You'd never even consider the prospect of going into battle alone, yet when it comes to fighting the battle of transition out of the military or first responder roles, many try to go it either alone or without the appropriate team surrounding them.

Just like in the military team environment, different people bring different *specialist* support to the transitioning individual. Also, just like in the military team environment, first and foremost is making sure that you are bringing the best version of yourself to the mission.

This means paying attention to your own personal wellbeing and optimising fundamentals such as sleep, nutrition, fitness, mindset, maintaining specialist skills, and knowledge of the operating environment.

Continuing to pay attention to these factors is especially important throughout the stress of the transition period to make sure you remain in the best physical and mental condition you can for the battle.

I'm not going to kick the arse out of how to optimise individual wellbeing here because we have done exactly that in the aforementioned book I co-authored *The Resilience Shield*. At the risk of shamelessly self-promoting, I recommend anyone negotiating the transition process give that one a read as well!

When it comes to other team members to fight the transition battle with, there are three main groups:

1. Tribe members
2. Family and friends, and
3. Mental health specialists.

Tribe Members

Tribe members are those who you feel understood by and who can viscerally empathise with the stress you are feeling. They are often people who have experienced the same stress as you, or something similar enough to know exactly how it makes you feel.

There's a real power in being surrounded by people who get it, and this is where a significant amount of social support can come from when an individual is part of the military or a first responder organisation.

As discussed in Chapter 4, what occurs on transition out of these roles is that you leave your tribe behind. You are no longer part of that in-group and by virtue of that fact, from the perspective of your former tribe, you are now a member of an out-group.

The problem is that most transitioning individuals will still *identify* as their former role for a significant period after leaving the job and will naturally want to reach back into their old tribe for support.

In my opinion this is akin to a young adult leaving home for the first time. If they're anything like me, they won't move far away and they'll often drop back home for the support of that familiar environment, not to mention to get a decent feed and have their clothes washed!

Over time however, they eventually find their feet living independently, build strong social supports outside of home, and visit their parents less and less. Their relationship with their parents hopefully remains strong, but it changes from one of being their sole support system when they were kids; to a significant support as young adults still living at home; to more of a peer support once they have become adults and left home.

The same needs to happen for a healthy transition out of military or first responder roles, with the relationship with the former tribe changing over time and relationships with new tribes forming.

When it comes to making sense of experiences that have happened during service in a former role, then the old tribe members might be uniquely positioned to provide support. I believe that tapping back into this old tribe is healthy to reminisce on the shared good experiences and any ongoing need to debrief some of the bad experiences along the way.

Caution needs to be exercised though that former tribe members are not the *only* support system for the transitioned member for too long post-transition. As to what defines too long, that's hard to say and will differ for everyone, but the point is that effort needs to be made to integrate into new tribes.

Given that the transitioning member is no longer part

of the old in-group, it's important to look at what new in-groups they are a part of. These can be the foundations of new tribes with people who can viscerally empathise with the individual's current stressors.

For instance, one new in-group that a transitioning military member will be a part of is the veteran in-group, and hence veteran organisations are a great place to find a new tribe. It's important to consider though that the tribal affiliation here needs to be formed around the shared experience of the group in transition to civilian life, and not exclusively trying to relate to one another based on their *previous* experience in uniform.

I have seen this process fail miserably when veterans fall into the trap of comparing their previous service and looking for similarities there to connect through. If those similarities exist then it can work well to bond the veterans, but often their service is so objectively different that no similarities are found and rather a competition can occur to establish some sort of perceived pecking order of whose service was *better* than the others'.

This can be avoided if the focus is instead placed on the shared challenges they are facing in the current, rather than those they faced in the past.

Do not fight the last war

A recurrent mantra that echoed throughout the training environment in my military days was:

Do not fight the last war.

The point being that we should always be future focused and looking at how best to prepare for success in the next war. As far as I can gather, this mantra comes from The Guerrilla War-Of-The-Mind Strategy cited in *The 33 Strategies of War* by Robert Greene[37], which in part reads:

> What often weighs you down and brings you misery is the past, in the form of unnecessary attachments, repetitions of tired formulas, and the memory of old victories and defeats. You must consciously wage war against the past and force yourself to react to the present moment. Be ruthless on yourself; do not repeat the same tired methods. Sometimes you must force yourself to strike out in new directions, even if they involve risk.

When fighting the war of transition, the tribe required is different from the one that suited the challenges of your old role.

As discussed in Chapter 12, it's important to start building new tribal bonds with people you share a future with, rather than those you shared a past with. This means *reacting* to the *present* and truly making the effort to connect and build relationships with new people you meet. While it often doesn't feel like it early in the transition process, with time and effort, a new sense of tribal affiliation can be found in a new workplace and social circles if you open your mind to the idea and embrace the change.

---

[37] Greene. R. *The 33 Strategies of War*. 2006. New York: Viking.

As discussed throughout this book, when I first discharged from the army, I felt completely isolated and disconnected from civilian society, but through throwing myself back into work as a doctor in the emergency department of a small hospital I found purpose, rebuilt my sense of self-worth, built a new identity, and integrated into a new tribe. It was only through shared experiences and hardships that I was able to forge this sense of tribe with my new workmates, and that took time and effort on my behalf.

One thing to bear in mind when finding new tribes is that you may never replicate the same sense of tribal affiliation that you did in the unique environment of the military or first response work. If you can, then great, but the objective is not necessarily to recreate *exactly* what you had in terms of social support and visceral understanding, but at a minimum to strive for human connection and group affiliation with people who share your current/future interests and the stressors unique to them.

Family and Friends

The necessary investment in military and first responder roles can come at the cost of time away from family and non-work friends. This is often compounded by the psychological distance that is created by unique exposures that can never be completely understood by those outside the role, and potentially the sense of distance created by operational security requirements that prevent the discussion of work-related events and information being shared outside of the work environment.

The transition period can often provide the time and opportunity to reconnect and re-establish or strengthen bonds with family and friends that might have been neglected over the years due to work commitments.

The key point to understand here is that your family and friends will never be able to truly *empathise* with the experiences you had in your former role and shouldn't be held accountable for this fact.

It took me quite some time to work that out with my wife!

During my time in uniform, I didn't tell my wife a lot about what I was up to. Part of it was due to operational security requirements, but mostly it was because I didn't want her to worry any more than necessary about me getting injured or worse. The fact that she had little to no interest in the army or my role within it helped tremendously with that!

It was only after discharge, when some of my unprocessed experiences came back to haunt me, that I first felt it might be useful to let my wife in on some of the key experiences I was trying to make sense of. At that point I decided to give her a somewhat watered-down version of an incident where I had responded to a teammate of mine who had struck an IED and who we had desperately tried to resuscitate for around 30 minutes, under complex conditions, before we eventually lost him.

As I told my wife the story, I could see that while she was

hearing the words, she didn't appear to be *getting it*.

She wasn't showing any of the emotional reactions that I felt were appropriate to the story.

Frustrated by this, I retold her the key parts of the story filling in all the vivid details and yet she still didn't appear to be getting it.

Initially this angered me, as if somehow she was diminishing or trivialising my experience. But after a couple of days, it finally occurred to me that it wasn't that she didn't *want* to get it, it was just that she simply *couldn't*. She had (thankfully) never had any experience even remotely like what I was trying to describe to her to be able to viscerally empathise with my experience. That certainly wasn't her fault, and therefore I certainly shouldn't have held her accountable.

The power of my relationship with my wife was that although she couldn't empathise with my experiences, I could be my authentic and vulnerable self in front of her, which I could never really be in front of my work tribe members. At the time of writing, she is the only person on Earth who I have cried in front of in the past 20 years, such is my ability to feel safe and be vulnerable around her.

It's essential to have some close family and friends in support of you during the transition process. Lean on them for the support of vulnerable and authentic relationships, but if they have never worked in the military or as a first responder, don't expect them to ever truly understand your experiences and be careful how much you share with them.

While it may seem useful to tell them vivid details of key experiences, you can risk traumatising them with the details, and it's unlikely that they'll be able to empathise anyway.

Mental health professionals and other specialist support

I've covered off on the unique skills of mental health professionals already in Chapter 14.

To reiterate briefly here, they are key specialist members of the optimised team to fight the transition battle with. They may not be able to empathise with your experiences like a tribe member would, and you may not be able to be completely authentic and vulnerable with them (at first at least) like you might with family and close friends, but they have the training and the evidence-based strategies to help you process past events and manage current stresses to help you power forward in life post-transition.

Psychologists and counsellors are the obvious go-to professionals in this category, however there is a wide range of professions that can help in this space. Having a good GP/Family Doctor in your corner is a powerful ally, as is a psychiatrist if required. Also on the list are Chaplains, Padres, and other religious and spiritual figures depending on your particular faith and affiliation.

The Trauma Processing Trident

Over the years since discharging from the army I have come to think of the optimal support structure to make sense of previous experiences and power forward in life as a trident model. I call it the *Trauma Processing Trident*.

Fundamental to the trident is the handle, which represents the individual *getting active in their own rescue* and proactively looking after their own wellbeing and resilience.

As illustrated in Figure 13, the prongs of the trident represent the three external support groups mentioned in this chapter:

1. Tribe members
2. Family and friends, and
3. Mental health professionals.

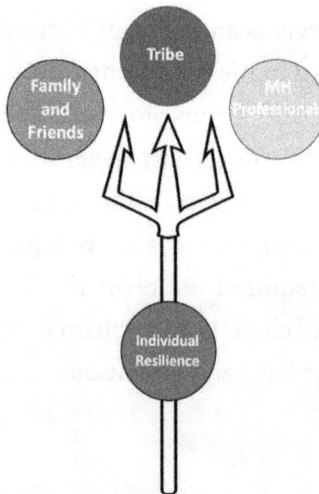

Figure 13. The Trauma Processing Trident

Call to Action: Build your Trident

The very final task in this book is to build your team to fight the next war with!

In the boxes below consider who is currently on, and who you would like to be on, your team in the various specialist positions. In the Individual Resilience boxes, write down all the things you are doing, or want to start doing, to *get active in your own rescue* to build and maintain the resilience you're going to need for the transition battle.

19. You can become relevant and consequential once more

The rock band Tool is my favourite band of all time and admittedly I probably read too deeply into the lyrics penned by their enigmatic singer Maynard James Keenan. That said, I find great relevance to a transitioning military member or first responder in the following lyrics from their song *Invincible*:

> Warrior struggling
> To remain relevant
> Warrior struggling
> To remain consequential

This pretty much sums up how I felt after I left the army; irrelevant and inconsequential.

At that point I found myself in a dark space where there was seemingly no way forward to a thriving version of myself and no way back to the formerly relevant and consequential version of myself.

My identity was firmly fused with the work role I had

left behind, I had abandoned my tribe, I was bored shitless, I was plagued by demons I could no longer outrun or supress with alcohol, I felt deeply isolated and lonely, and I lacked purpose and motivation.

Fast forward to now and I can honestly say that I am thriving. I once more feel relevant, consequential, and self-actualised. I am again the best version of myself, and I have found my new ikigai.

The path was not always clear and there have been many dark days. During the times of darkness, I tried to remind myself that I didn't need to illuminate the entire path forward. On some days I stumbled further backwards into the darkness. On other days, casting a dim light on a single step forward was enough.

The content of this book has come from nearly a decade of negotiating my path out of the darkness. It is the book that I wished I had been handed during my initial failed encounter with the psychologist following discharge.

As mentioned in the introduction, this book is the shit that I wished I knew before I discharged, and I appreciate that the entirety of its contents may not resonate with every reader. All our paths will differ, so take from this book what resonates with you and is useful to form the foundations of your own path, and then get active in building the rest.

If you're reading this book, you are not broken.

You have been a thriving version of yourself in the past and you can become that again. You have skills and experience that the world can benefit from. You will be carrying trauma, but I encourage you to view it as a fuel. It can either burn your house down in the form of Post-Traumatic Stress, or it can warm you in the form of Post Traumatic Growth. Find the right professional support and look hard for the silver linings to the dark trauma clouds as this is where the growth can be found.

Know that your transition to a positive new identity will take years, not months. Be kind to yourself during the process.

Remember the sage words of Matthew McConaughey:

"Once you know it's black, it's not near as dark"

Transition is a black space; I truly hope that this book helps enlighten it for you and I wish you every success in life post military or first responder service.

Thank you all for what you have done for your countries and communities.

20. About the author

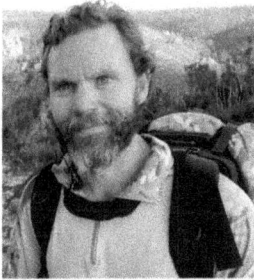

Dan Pronk had a profoundly average Australian upbringing, the son of an army helicopter pilot father and speech therapist mother, he had one brother and a cat growing up. After attending seven schools and getting expelled from one, he graduated high school with average grades and began the ambitious pursuit of a career in professional triathlon. Five years later when that failed, on a whim he applied for the army and sat the entrance test for medical school, being successful in both and setting him on a trajectory to becoming an army doctor.

A year later and encounter with a group of army Special Operations soldiers led to a lightbulb moment for Dan, he *had* to join Special Operations and be part of what they do. The only problem was it would be six years before he would be allowed on the selection course for the Australian Special Air Service Regiment (SASR). Undeterred, Dan set his sights on selection and year-in, year-out bettered himself with a view to completing selection. In 2008 Dan successfully completed the SASR selection course and went on to become one of Australia's most highly deployed and decorated Special Operations doctors.

After five years with Special Operations Dan discharged to pursue a career in civilian medicine, as well as further study in the form of a Master of Business Administration. Demons from Dan's military time would catch up with him after discharge and following a period of struggle with symptoms of Post-Traumatic Stress, he emerged out the other side a stronger person, experiencing Post Traumatic Growth.

Post-army Dan has gone on to hold leadership roles in hospitals and state-wide medical services, to co-own a multimillion dollar company, and to found a number of entrepreneurial startups. Dan is the bestselling author of multiple books including his autobiography *The Combat Doctor*, as well as *The Resilience Shield*, which he co-authored with two fellow SAS veterans, and uses the author's collective reflections, as well as a deep dive into the contemporary literature on stress and resilience, to present resilience as a dynamic, multifactorial, and modifiable construct that we can all deliberately and proactively build.

Dan has worked as the on-set doctor for reality TV shows including SAS Australia and Alone and stays engaged with tactical medicine as an instructor and advisor for military and police tactical elements and as the Medical Director for the private company TacMed Australia.

He lives in South Australia with his very tolerant wife and his three sons and can often be found driving his vintage Lamborghini in the Adelaide Hills, or standing next to it on the side of the road waiting for yet another tow truck when it regularly breaks down.

21. More from Dan

The Combat Doctor

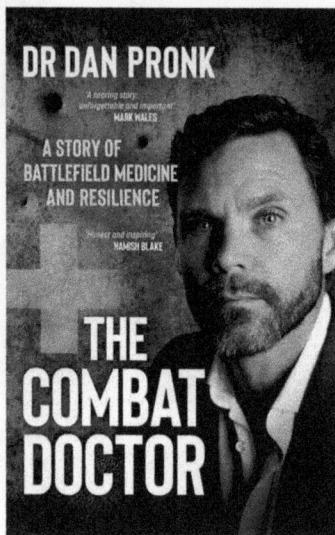

'I had seen dozens of people die horrible deaths ... This time was different. This time it was a friend of mine dying in the dirt in front of me, and it was my job to save him.'

Dr Dan Pronk served on over 100 combat missions in Afghanistan as a frontline special forces combat doctor, where the casualties he treated were his fellow SAS soldiers and commandos, local civilians and even the enemy.

The thrill of adventure and the challenges of battlefield medicine brought out the very best in Dan; he discovered a sense of purpose in pushing his medical skills and courage to the limits. But there was a cost.

In this frank and vivid memoir, Dan describes the highs and lows of his military-medical career, and the very real toll they took on his mental health and family life. He writes movingly about the burden of saving - and failing to save - friends and comrades, the feelings of helplessness and despair that haunted him, and the journey back to a meaningful and fulfilling civilian life.

The *Combat Doctor* is an extraordinary story of resilience and growth, and a tribute to the doctors and medics working behind the scenes in conflict around the world.

Praise for *The Combat Doctor*

'I love Dan's insight from his beginnings as an everyday guy, who pushes himself into operating in a very, very non-everyday environment. A fascinating account of what it is like to go into battle, and the unseen mental battles that arise from the experience. Honest and inspiring. I loved it.'
- Hamish Blake

'Dr Pronk walks us to the very gates of hell and points to the nightmare that is modern warfare. The thrall of combat, the dread of buried mines, and the shattered bodies of his mates all feature in this parallel universe that was Australia's war in Afghanistan. This is not some well-worn trope of heroism in war - it brings to life the ghosts of Australia's best fighters: their grit, their humour, and their final moments. These fallen sons both haunted and inspired Dan to live a complete life. A searing story: unforgettable and important.'
- Mark Wales

'Beyond the headlines, popular imagery and mythology of SAS and Commandos, are stories of duty and devotion to one another. The Combat Doctor is both a participant and an observer - of skill, courage, death and growth from the traumatic aftermath of war. Step out of your comfort zone, accept the challenge to a better person.' - Dr Brendan Nelson

'Dr Dan Pronk transports the reader into the boots and under the combat helmet of Special Forces in a way few writers can. The idea of a fully armed doctor engaging with an enemy to potentially take life and then within seconds fighting to save one is an incredibly unique perspective. Dan's memoir of his time as a combat doctor, saving lives and at times losing them in the midst of battle, offers a rare, heartfelt perspective of the best, bravest and worst of humanity - but one we all benefit from hearing. ' - Merrick Watts

'Dan gives us an uncensored look into the darkest sides of combat and a raw, personal account of events that have become legend in the Special Forces world. An open, frank look into the mind of the doctor you want by your side when the unthinkable happens.' - Damien Thomlinson

The Resilience Shield
(co-authored with Ben Pronk and Tim Curtis)

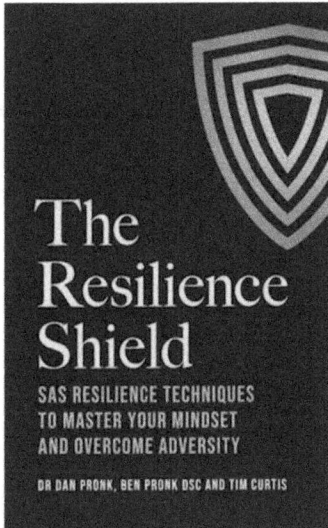

'a powerful text that will benefit any reader' - Dr Richard Harris SC, OAM, hero of the Thai cave rescue

Life is hard. Rocketing rates of physical and mental health issues are testimony to the immense pressures of our complex world. So how do we become tough and adaptable to face life's challenges?

The Resilience Shield provides that defence. In their groundbreaking guide to overcoming adversity, Australian SAS veterans Dr Dan Pronk, Ben Pronk DSC and Tim Curtis take you behind the scenes of special operations missions, into the boardrooms of leading companies and through the depths of contemporary research in order to demystify and define resilience. Through lessons learned in and out of uniform, they've come to understand the critical components of resilience and how it can be developed in anyone - including you.

The Resilience Shield explores the hard-won resilience secrets of elite soldiers and the latest thinking on mental and physical wellbeing. This book will equip you with an arsenal of practical tools for you to start making immediate improvements in your life that are attainable and sustainable.

Let's build your shield!

Praise for *The Resilience Shield*

'informative and enlightening . . . compelling lessons and advice' - The Hon Julie Bishop

'Clear, approachable insights into resilience' - Merrick Watts

'A blend of raw experience and impeccable science...a brilliant guidebook for our times' - Hugh Mackay AO

Average 70kg D**khead

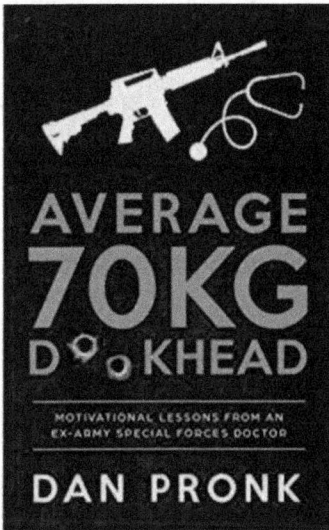

Ever get the feeling that you're destined for great things, but you don't quite know how to get started? Perhaps you're stuck in a rut with life passing you by and a fear that you will die wondering what you could have achieved? If so this book is for you.

*Average 70kg D**khead* tracks key life events of Dr Dan Pronk from his beginnings as an average chubby kid, through his failed attempt at professional triathlon, onto becoming a doctor, joining army Special Forces, being decorated for his conduct in action in Afghanistan, and then onto his post-army career as a medical executive and co-owner of a multimillion dollar business.

Throughout the book Dan shares his motivational philosophies and key lessons learned from his journey. He breaks down the goal setting process and provides examples of how seemingly impossible goals can be deconstructed into smaller and smaller achievable sub-goals, creating a clear pathway to getting started and moving towards your ambitious objectives.

Dan highlights the crucial factor of persistence in goal attainment and uses case studies from the Special Forces selection process to illustrate that average people with above-average persistence will beat stronger, smarter, faster, and more educated people who are not as willing to persist every time.

This book will inspire you to do more. Be it to get off the couch and get started, or double down on your existing goals and supercharge your commitment to them. You only get one go at this life, so what are you waiting for? Give it a read and get going!

www.ingramcontent.com/pod-product-compliance
Lightning Source LLC
Chambersburg PA
CBHW031157270326
41931CB00006B/309